PANIC ATTACK

Also by Nicole Saphier

Make America Healthy Again

PANIC ATTACK

PLAYING POLITICS WITH
SCIENCE IN THE FIGHT
AGAINST COVID-19

NICOLE SAPHIER

BROADSIDE BOOKS
An Imprint of HarperCollinsPublishers

HarperCollins books may be purchased for educational, business, or sales promotional use. For information, please email the Special Markets Department at SPsales@harpercollins.com.

Broadside Books™ and the Broadside logo are trademarks of HarperCollins Publishers.

FIRST EDITION

Library of Congress Cataloging-in-Publication Data has been applied for.

ISBN 978-0-06-307969-4

21 22 23 24 25   LSC   10 9 8 7 6 5 4 3 2 1

This book was written in honor of the frontline workers, who despite the tumultuous landscape and plethora of misinformation, continued to work tirelessly during the COVID-19 crisis.

We pass through this world but once. Few tragedies can be more extensive than the stunting of life, few injustices deeper than the denial of an opportunity to strive or even to hope, by a limit imposed from without, but falsely identified as lying within.

—STEPHEN JAY GOULD

CONTENTS

INTRODUCTION

At this point, we are all so used to having to wash our hands many times a day, put on masks, and practice social distancing that it sometimes feels as though COVID-19 has been around forever. A colleague recently remarked to me that when he watches old television series, he finds himself worrying that the characters in the show are standing too close to one another. Just as the buildings in New York City are classified as prewar versus postwar, it would seem television shows, and all things as we have known them, are soon to be known as pre-COVID and post-COVID.

If you turn on the car radio, it is hard to escape nonstop talk about the virus. The same goes for social media. All of this dialogue would be great if it were all accurate. Unfortunately, much of the conversation is grounded in rumors and, you guessed it—panic. Accusations, rhetoric, and paranoid doomsday scenarios are mingled in with facts. It is sometimes hard to tell what is real and what is not.

Of all the words that we most commonly hear these days in the wake of the pandemic, perhaps the most pervasive and powerful are those that have to do with *fear*. People are understandably afraid—for their children's futures, for their own lives, for the most vulnerable among us, and for our future as Americans.

Lurking within the fear is anger, and anger, as most of us know from experience, comes with a desire to assign blame—something or someone to be designated as the source of our pain.

The anger is not limited to domestic foes, as there is also anger toward the Chinese Communist government for concealment of information, and allowing infected people to travel internationally after it was known that the virus was being transmitted among humans.

Understandably, there is anger about the ensuing loss of life—about the anguish of senior citizens dying alone from direct orders by predominantly Democratic governors. Anger for children being tossed aside by partisan politics and the legislators responsible who caved to political pressure and ignored all childhood health experts. All the while, these people were claiming to *follow the science*.

There is anger about the authoritarian shutdown of businesses, and the destruction of the American Dream for millions of Americans, despite science saying otherwise. Not to mention the fallout from universal financial insecurity, with many under the pressure of lockdown succumbing to addictions that they had previously overcome or the emergence of new mental and physical health maladies.

Panic Attack is what happens when one party declares they are the party of science and then assumes everything they want to be true is now scientific.

Many measures enforced by politicians everywhere, with the majority being Democratic, ignored common sense and scientific data as they shut down beaches, playgrounds, and National Parks while allowing Big Business to remain open. Governor Gretchen Whitmer banned the purchase of seeds, a purchase that would have encouraged people to be outdoors instead of inside in poorly ventilated spaces. People were allowed to continue packing the Goliath mega-stores yet unable to jog alone on a path without wearing a mask.

Through the stories of these and other unscientific policies, I will explore two ideas. The first is about how experts make their recommendations. The same qualities that give experts their strength—their certainty over complicated things—turn out to also be their greatest weakness. Their lack of transparency, appeals to authority, and poor science communication made their advice seem arbitrary, high-handed, and pointless.

The entire mantra that a single political party was *following the science* while the other was not was wiped away over the course of the pandemic as the hypocrisy of "do what I say, not what I do" played out in various avenues while Americans everywhere were suffering.

Some of this comes from experts telling us their conclusions without explaining how they got there. Much of it comes from politicians cherry-picking the expert conclusions they want. As a society, we consistently get these conflicts that support their chosen agenda. We misread who the conflict is among. We misinterpret what the expert consensus is. We get lost when two experts we trust seem to be saying opposite things. If they can't explain, we can't understand.

Resentment has grown from how American public discourse has changed since the unprecedented events of 2020 began. More specifically, people are angry about the fact that, these days, it seems only one set of opinions is allowed. If they deviate, if they question, they are defectors. More than that, by virtue of being defectors, they are *de facto* deplorables, who should be denounced, fired, and canceled. *We shouldn't have to explain anything*, politicians said. *Because we are right.*

So-called progressives, like the rest of us, sometimes judge based on opinions rather than knowledge, especially when we feel fear. Except, part of being a citizen of a constitutional, democratic republic is that each of us—and all of us, collectively—have the right and the opportunity to use our own reason to move beyond opinions, through experiment, to facts and truth. We can pursue the truth individually and jointly. Through that pursuit, we can acquire knowledge, and knowledge, as the 17th-century philosopher Francis Bacon once stated, is power. In our current moment, power seems to lie in stirring up fear. We need, then, to recover a different, more constructive kind of power—the power inherent in truth. No single person owns the truth. It belongs to everyone.

When pundits, experts, and legislators alike denied, or at least downplayed, the growing humanitarian crisis caused by the pandemic response as not being real or scientifically measurable, faith in them was lost by those who were living through it. It's not surprising the populace wants to hear more than "Trust us" when life is on the line.

To be sure, we face obstacles. Among these obstacles are false, self-proclaimed prophets, who strive to weaponize people's fears and then manipulate those worries to secure support for themselves or their YouTube videos or other platform. These individuals may use real experts' mistakes as proof of their own "expertise." The bottom line is, any critic can find something to confirm their own individual narrative. The great advances in life are not made primarily or exclusively through our own aggrandizement while criticizing others. Don't get me wrong—it's important to practice critical thinking and not blindly toe the line, with respect to both our own opinions and those of others. Thus, an open dialogue of conflicting opinion under the auspices of mutual regard and transparency is the only way for a civilized society to be unified.

The problem is, most experts do not spend time preparing to see their work abused by Twitter reply guys or their big-city mayor. This is never the battle they expect to fight. Experts are great at providing information—they're not great at communicating it in ways that prevent power-hungry and panicked politicians from using that information to achieve partisan goals.

Which brings me to my second point: the politicizing of science makes the job of scientific discovery much harder. Not only does it influence important research, but it can also close off important deliberations on the outcomes. As the normal process, mixed with nefarious intentions, unfolded in front of the public eye, the entire course undermined public faith in science when the politics influencing it turned out to be wrong. Not to mention, while there is merit to clinical trials, we became increasingly aware of the endless suffering and excess death occurring from regulatory inaction and political influence.

Over the course of this book, I'm going to come back to this again and again. Partisanship has led people to think they have all the answers when what they really should have are questions. We must be prepared to follow where the science leads. We shouldn't assume our preconceived political beliefs will always be supported by science. As Sherlock Holmes would put it: we should never theorize in advance of the facts.

The best sources for truth are those who can admit with all due humility that they don't have all the information when it is lacking and acknowledge their biases when pointing to a source.

The physicist Richard Feynman famously kept a notebook, on the first page of which he wrote:

NOTEBOOK OF THINGS I DON'T KNOW ABOUT.

He knew that inquiry begins not with an inventory of what we DO know, but with awareness of and curiosity about what we DON'T know. Those of us who understand we lack information are willing to take a risk to go above and beyond what is not known and, if we find something new, to let knowledge of it flourish. Pride must not get in the way.

Our American temperament is grounded in the notion that our country is itself an experiment—an experiment, as noted by Alexander Hamilton in *Federalist Papers* No. 1, as to whether "societies of men are really capable or not of establishing good government from reflection and choice or whether they are forever destined to depend for their political constitutions on accident and force."

Despite the best and even noble efforts of so many, the overall landscape of COVID-19 has been dominated by accident and force, rather than reflection and choice. It is overwhelmed by fear, panic, personal ambition, and anger. As a result, the knowledge of

facts—and the pursuit of truth that relies upon facts as its basis—
is at risk.

The information driving the crisis response and that which is
being conveyed on television by reputable reporters and contributors is largely based on information from preprints, observational
studies, and opinion pieces. As a result, it's difficult for the public
to understand the difference between legitimate, data-driven science and that which is equivalent to anecdotal reports informed
merely by a desire to share preliminary knowledge or, regrettably, to make a sensation. This ultimately allows people who don't
know what they are doing to cherry-pick data and use it to support their own agenda, all in the name of science. It also creates
a vacuum of confusion and apprehension when the preliminary
information is subsequently determined to be wrong.

Public health experts and elected officials, as well as the Centers for Disease Control and Prevention (CDC) and the World
Health Organization (WHO), have demonstrated both strengths
and weaknesses.

At the end of the day, whichever way you look at it, many actions
taken initially will be deemed mistakes retrospectively. No one will be
satisfied with the way that everything about the situation is handled.

We are so busy fighting with one another that sometimes we lose
sight of the fact that the real bad guy is the virus itself. In other
words, we must stop the infighting and work together to eradicate
this pathogen to maintain being a prosperous society.

That does not mean, however, that we need to throw up our
hands and say "everybody makes mistakes; let's just move on," or
that we can merely ask, along with the author of an op-ed in *The
New York Times*, "Can we please just blame the virus?" To whatever extent possible, we need to assign responsibility and assume
accountability where appropriate. But the domain of responsibility
does not and should not entail demonization and humiliation, nor
should any measures be taken for personal gain at the expense of
others.

Proud people are having to ask for government assistance, and millions who worked in the service industry relying on tips are now on unemployment. There are countless people we will never hear about whose lives have been shattered by despair, loneliness, and suicide.

The most promising way out of this trap of blaming and shaming lies in the responsible pursuit of truth. We need to move forward together, armed with the knowledge necessary to make educated, informed decisions, aimed at protecting ourselves, our family, and our fellow Americans. We also need to hold our elected and non-elected leaders liable for mishaps while demanding better preparedness and response for future calamities.

Because they will come.

If the public has learned a lesson from COVID-19, it is that science oftentimes does not generate certainty and that the overall health of a nation rarely hangs on a single facet of a complex truth. We are still acquiring and processing the facts about SARS-CoV-2, the virus responsible for the pandemic, and will be for a while. True, we seem to have gotten past the worst of it, but we need to take a step back and evaluate what we know and consider what we don't—and may never—know so we are prepared for any future surges.

To do this, we must do two things. We must not politicize the science. A disappointing occurrence is that scientific data from the world's leading experts regarding the novel coronavirus has been constantly distorted to fit politically motivated narratives. Mixed messages are everywhere. Who should and can we trust? We need transparent science we can all trust.

And to that end, we need experts and politicians to explain their reasoning—not just tell us what to do. The United States is not short of experts to assess and advise the country's response to the crisis. A benefit of having so many experts is that they can explain science to the public in an understandable format. Yet, an expert saying "just do this" only convinces the already convinced, and when more people are engaging in social media discussions rather than heeding the words of the specialists, something has gone wrong. Misinformation spread during the pandemic from the misinformed who did a better job of explaining their side, or who were relying on political kinsmanship to keep from having to explain it. Still, even when information is misconstrued, censorship without transparent discussion only makes it worse, especially when followed by experts saying "this is wrong so move on."

The chaos has unveiled the reality that even our top authorities have moments in which they have to say, "I don't know." Yet people are so desperate for certainty—and for weapons to beat up their opponents and rivals—that we end up glued to social media and hanging on every last word as if someone, somewhere, has the secret key to knowledge—often distorted to fit their own belief.

This book tries to see past the panic. It conveys the facts as best it can, as seen through the lens of medical research, expertise, and experience. We were told to *follow the science*, but it seems a once objective scientific path became subjective and widely open to manipulation, abuse, and misinformation. Here we will try to connect the facts to the truth and, beyond that, our goals for the future.

PANIC ATTACK

CHAPTER 1

POLITICIZING SCIENCE AT THE EXPENSE OF THE PEOPLE

August 12, 2020, was not the hottest day of the summer in Wilmington, Delaware. It was only in the mid-80s at its peak. It was, however, quite sticky—verging at points in the late afternoon on uncomfortably humid. It made sense, then, that the kickoff for the newly united Democratic ticket for president and vice president of the United States—comprising former Vice President Joe Biden and Senator Kamala Harris—took place not in the heat of the outdoors, but in the almost empty gymnasium of A. I. du Pont High School in Greenville, Delaware.

Harris, as expected, wasted no time in attacking her political opponent on the grounds that he had destroyed the economy. Had she been named as the candidate for vice president prior to the outbreak of SARS-CoV-2, of course, her opening remarks would have fallen flat. Prior to the pandemic, the American economy was roaring ahead. But in the wake of the lockdown, as most American readers know, the picture was very different.

Not only did Harris lambaste the current administration for forcing the economy into ruin, she also attempted to indict it for an incompetent response to the pandemic. She sought to contrast

President Trump's response to SARS-CoV-2 to the reaction of then-President Obama for the 2013 Ebola outbreak.

The Ebola crisis, of course, was nothing like the COVID-19 pandemic. But a lack of facts did not stop the deriding by Harris. In her account, one administration—representing that of the party with which she is allied—did brilliantly in handling the threat of a dangerous disease while the other—representing the party that she opposes—did horribly. Harris went so far as to falsely imply Ebola, like SARS-CoV-2—was a pandemic. "Six years ago, in fact, we had a different health crisis," Harris said. "It was called Ebola. We all remember that pandemic."

Indeed, we do not—since Ebola was not a pandemic and there are more dissimilarities between the two public health emergencies than actual similarities. Had Senator Harris or her speechwriters consulted the World Health Organization website or learned a minuscule amount about virology and public health, the distinction between an outbreak and a pandemic, as well as the stark transmissibility differences between SARS-CoV-2 and Ebolavirus, would have been readily evident. But accuracy was not really the point. Scoring political points through bombastic statements under the guise of "science," whether they were correct or not, was the goal.

Politicizing science for talking points ultimately undermines public faith in science, especially when the politicians speaking about it are in fact wrong. It didn't take long in the pandemic for the process to start, for after an initial showing of unity when the novel coronavirus entered our borders, people in the United States divided over basic scientific facts about COVID-19.

At the beginning of the crisis, people were mostly united. We trusted what science and government told us—and what government told us the science was. We were all in it together, Republican and Democrat.

Eventually the phrase "follow the science" became one of the most divisive messaging campaigns of the period. Truthfully, most people believed they were following the science and doing what was best for them and those around them. Unfortunately, recommendations and data were changing constantly, nothing was consistent, and misinformation ran rampant.

Once the pandemic gained footing in the United States, conflicting messages flooded a panicking public. Some of the people spreading lies had political motivations, like the Chinese Communist Party providing inaccurate information about the virus, while whistleblower accounts from medical personnel were stifled. In the United States, Democratic hopefuls criticized any moves by the Trump administration as "failures." Some people, domestic and foreign, attempted to make a profit on sham miracle cures, while others were trying to increase their media presence and academic clout.

Throughout all of this, the collective emotional response was filtered through a rosy view of scientists as the white knights who would shepherd us through this trial. One popular misconception, though, is that scientists are, by definition, altruistic figures devoted solely to the pursuit of objective truth.

Science is immune to politics, in this line of thinking, because it subjects claims to the rigors of experimental proof and deep theoretical exploration. Scientists, therefore, are egalitarian saints, who would never be led astray by the wish to promote their careers or political commitments. We should never question them. We should simply "have faith in science" and dismiss any others who give contrarian advice as being corrupt stooges and even bad scientists to boot.

But science, of course, is as fallible as any other field, and subject to the political biases of its practitioner. One only has to remember the rise and fall of Soviet biologist Trofim Lysenko to understand why there is a movement questioning government control on the basis of *science*. Lysenko famously, or rather infamously, rejected traditional Mendelian genetics and proposed an alternate to farming crops, called vernalization. His method proposed fertilizing fields without traditional fertilizers and minerals while being less costly and able to produce more robust crops, providing a solution to the agriculture crisis the country was facing in the 1930s. He went to the government with his solution, and given the crisis on hand, no one thought to verify his claims.

Lysenko was portrayed as a genius and became skillful at denouncing his scientific opponents who failed at reproducing his claims on the basis of not *following the science*. He used surveys from farmers to prove that vernalization increased crop yields, thus avoiding any controlled tests of his methods. Ultimately, years of famine and poor crop production led to millions of people starving to death at the hands of a scientist who made claims that could not be substantiated through controlled trials, and who got political support for it, perverting science through politics and misleading populations under the guise of *following the science*.

Nearly a century later, Americans are caught in the middle of controlling a pandemic with methods being drawn from the support of politicians, scientists, and even Hollywood celebrities. As with Lysenko, legislation is being passed and local directives are put forth in the name of science with limited evidence, and with critics being censored and demeaned as *anti-science*.

Once more, there are actions being taken without being backed by facts or science. Many claim to *follow the science*, but they're really just using this charade of intellectual and moral superiority to justify harsh restrictions. And once more, the fact that many people are suffering is disregarded as the overall cause is alleged to be more important than other human consequences.

As regulatory standards, treatment discovery, mask-wearing, and even the number of confirmed infections were being aggressively politicized, two narratives materialized dominating the discourse about SARS-CoV-2, both being grounded in politics under the guise of the pursuit of science. The first narrative was that Democrats were noble public servants, intrepidly *following the science*, in every particular of their many lockdown regulations. The other narrative, of course, was that anyone who complained about Democrat policies was, therefore, anti-science, no matter how well-reasoned their objections.

How did the commentary develop that, with respect to SARS-CoV-2, one political party became known as pro-science and the other anti-science? We might certainly read this phenomenon as just another chapter in the popular representation of Republicans being anti-science conspiracy theorists and Democrats as oppressive socialists, but that doesn't really explain how regulatory standards, testing, and even immunity have come to serve as grounds for political warfare in the context of the pandemic. The reality is that the "science" we got was often contradictory, confusing, and sometimes, straight up wrong. This wasn't always scientists' faults—being wrong or uncertain about a mystery disease is normal and serves as the impetus behind trial-and-error experimentation. But politicians would often, once they were committed to a course of action, refuse to reverse course even when new scientific data showed they should. This broke the fragile trust that the crisis had forged between Americans of different beliefs.

Feeling they couldn't trust official science, many Americans turned to pseudoscience. As the pandemic continued playing out, it was no surprise when the development of a controversial video promoting an alternate theory became widely shared and promoted on social media platforms: "Plandemic"—a video full of hoax theories highlighting a disgraced former researcher who spoke disparagingly about the nation's health experts, the CDC, and vaccines. The production even suggested Dr. Anthony Fauci of the National Institutes of Health intentionally released the virus in an effort to kill people. The video went "viral" because by that point, people needed to identify an adversary and assign blame, despite the lack of evidence for the accusations. The video itself followed the blueprint of every conspiracy theory: a proposed philosophy in contradiction to the commonly accepted explanation, suspicion of official accounts (CDC, WHO), allegations of nefarious intentions by such officials, and victimization of the conspirators. Unfortunately, it's nearly impossible to change a conspiracy theorist's mind because their philosophies have become solidified and self-referential. The basic lack of evidence for such theories further adds to the "evidence" of a cover-up. The concepts therefore become immune to contradictory evidence because any scientific evidence provided that doesn't fit into the narrative must be falsified. This, of course, undermines medical workers and expert scientists, causing massive suspicion of any subsequent public health recommendations.

Trust continued to fade as Americans started voting in the 2020 presidential election.

It is hard to imagine anyone naïve enough to think that the 2020 presidential election cycle would *not* hinge upon the politicization of SARS-CoV-2. At this point, we have become so used to scientific results, standards, and even data being manipulated that it may seem hard to even react to this problem or to imagine that things could be otherwise. We have come to expect that one political party will devoutly claim it "believes in science" (a somewhat ironic claim since it posits following science as an object of faith) and that the other believes only in God, guns, and limited government. Both portraits, needless to say, are based upon hyperbole.

The pandemic has affected every American and has caused so much pain for so many people that it was irresistibly attractive for politicians on both sides of the aisle to weaponize it. Politicians thrive on the principle that one should never let a crisis go to waste. Thus, it's not hard to see why this has become the case.

Politicians hope to blame their opponent for a disaster and the pain it has caused, and to represent themselves as the means of resolving the calamity and bringing prosperity back to the nation.

"Vote for me and I will make all of your troubles disappear."

Isn't that what all campaigning politicians tell us? Clearly the tactic isn't new; in fact we have been seeing it our entire lives.

The easiest way to convince the public of their need to vote for you is to cast your opponent as an object of fear, and yourself as a means of relieving that fear. What greater opportunity than during a pandemic coinciding with a presidential election year to manipulate the fear of the public to get elected? If you have to distort science, so what?

There's a lot of political opportunity in turning every single public health directive into a partisan issue, which should then be debated to death by talk show hosts and YouTubers and politicians cynically wishing to cast the other side as the villains. The danger, of course, is that in the absence of consistent and sound messaging from the top down, the ability to rely on voluntary compliance of public health measures shrinks. So much of public health is about relying on individuals to make voluntary choices. People get confused and rebellious when they perceive politicians to simply be pushing "science" that's suspiciously similar to those politicians' previously stated policy objectives. Politicizing science erodes trust at a moment when voluntary actions of following public health directives is vital.

Clearly, it is much easier to force entities rather than individuals to change behaviors. Unfortunately, the political about-face and harsh measures rebuffed entire communities, and convinced few, if any, to change their minds or their ways.

Tragedies allow people to form communities by identifying villains and heroes, and subsequently allowing us to reject the former and rally around the latter. It can be consoling to be part of a group allied against a clearly evil rogue, even if the villain and hero are the products of partisan distortion. With respect to real-life struggles, the idea that there are heroes and villains battling it out who need our support enhances morale and helps us to endure sacrifices in the spirit of, to use the British idiom, "doing our bit" as part of a larger effort.

The ideal of everyone pitching in to a collective effort, to a large extent, is wonderful and, indeed, necessary as we are social creatures. The problem is that when a common effort is viewed through the lens of a crisis, we tend to see only heroes in our allies and villains as anyone contrarian, leading us to potentially hinder progress, and forgo tolerance of our fellow Americans.

The other threat, of course, is that we will pretend that there is no crisis at all, pretending all is normal, and thereby possibly harming or even fatally exposing others and ourselves to hazards.

We might call these two stances the "Toe the Line" approach where one lines up and acts accordingly without challenge, and the "Head in the Sand" approach where one is stubbornly unwilling to acknowledge an unpleasantry.

Neither approach is the best way to view public health emergencies. For one thing, either style raises the risk that, caught up in our enthusiasm to defeat the enemy, we will turn everything into weapons—including scientific research and data—to push our narrative. One of the most difficult things that can be done is trying to explain to someone why something would work when that person hasn't committed to making "it" work.

The weaponization of everything in the quest of victory is not a phenomenon that came into play with the spread of SARS-CoV-2, of course. It is a tendency of human nature. When politicians get involved, this tendency—creating "evils" particular to either political party—results in the politicization of science.

Indeed, such politicization is a weakness of the American project, which was itself envisioned by the founders as an "experiment" as to whether human beings could live on the basis of reflection and choice rather than the passions arising from accident and force.

When science—along with its regulatory standards and results—becomes politically influenced, we risk abandoning the American experiment and reverting to government control out of fear.

As it turned out in 2020, misinformation about the pandemic led to a second emergency: a profound underlying emergency of panic across America.

CHAPTER 2

WIDESPREAD PANIC

In 1918, the United States government mirrored the same communications approach to address the flu pandemic that it had developed to spread war news—which is to say, an optimistic view of the fight, spun to make the government look good. President Woodrow Wilson disdained the ability of citizens to make decisions in the crisis, and instructed that government communication must be focused on maintaining morale.

However, it was not ordinary influenza as they had experienced in the past. "The disease was unusual enough to be misdiagnosed initially," John M. Barry wrote in a 2009 *Nature* article, with the new influenza being mistaken for diseases far more deadly like "cholera, typhoid and dengue," and some people dying within 24 hours of the first symptom. Barry continues: "The most horrific feature was bleeding, not just from the nose and mouth but also from the ears and eyes," making people believe this was a more harrowing illness such as a hemorrhagic fever or even the plague.

"Nonetheless, the government and newspapers continued to reassure," writes Barry.

In Philadelphia, for example, public-health director Wilmer Krusen promised—before a single civilian had died—to "confine this disease to its present limits. In this we are sure to be successful." As the death toll grew, he repeatedly reassured the public that "the disease has about reached its crest. The situation is well in hand." When the number of daily deaths broke 200, he again promised: "The peak of the epidemic has been reached." When 300 died in a day, he said: "These deaths mark the high-water mark." Ultimately, daily deaths reached 759. The press never questioned him. . . . Unfortunately, Philadelphia's communication strategy was the rule, not the exception.

Yet, exceptional communication tactics in certain localities led to improved outcomes and improved public awareness. It became apparent that when people were provided accurate information to counter the challenges they were faced with, they often performed better, as they were not paralyzed in a panic from a lack of communication. Barry continues:

In San Francisco, for example, despite a slow reaction to the initial onslaught of flu, in October 1918 the mayor, health officials and business and union leaders all signed a full-page newspaper advert in huge type reading: "Wear A Mask and Save Your Life!" It was a rare, bold statement. In this city, society, although reeling, functioned. Food was delivered, and the sick were cared for. Where people had accurate information and knew what they faced, they often performed heroically. Red Cross professionals, physicians, and nurses routinely risked their lives. When Philadelphia's city police—who knew the facts even if the papers weren't printing them—were asked to supply four volunteers to "remove bodies from beds . . . and load them in vehicles," 118 officers responded.

As the contagious illness made its way across the country, quarantine and isolation measures were swiftly executed. Daily reports of increasing hospitalization and death counts circulated, while information being reported from "credible" sources pushing the government line was found to be unreliable. The mixed messaging with social isolation quickly took its toll as political tensions began to intensify. Americans began not only questioning public health recommendations but rejecting them, asserting their right to work and provide for their families. Neighbors were turning on each other as long-standing social injustices and riots broke out. If this sounds familiar, it should; while the same scenario has played out over the course of our global history of pandemics, it is occurring now as a result of COVID-19.

As Barry concludes, "The truth should not be managed, it should be told. Only by knowing the truth can imaginary horrors be transformed into concrete realities. And only then can people start to deal with those realities, and do so without panic."

THE CONDITIONS AND CONTAGION OF PANIC

Dispatch from the front lines: I'm now seeing people of all political persuasions in our psychiatric clinic, who genuinely believe the Apocalypse is near. Literally. And I'm not talking about individuals who are psychotic or manic. Otherwise healthy people are terrified.

This tweet, posted by California psychiatrist Dr. Aaron Kheriaty in late September 2020, echoed what countless doctors and mental health professionals have seen throughout the pandemic. The people showing up for treatment were not just the "worried well"—which is what people who "are anxious about their health, unwilling to accept reassurance, demanding investigation and referrals" are often called—but also people whose precarious conditions, such as anxiety, had tipped over into becoming more severe by exposure to a series of severe stressors.

The year 2020, as we all know, did not lack for immediate and distant stressors, both large and small.

The year began with raging fires in Australia. The fires were extinguished as the pandemic exploded, leading to lockdown and economic chaos. The deaths of George Floyd and Breonna Taylor generated peaceful protests, but also riots and chaos. Nature then unleashed hurricanes, as irresponsible users of fireworks and arsonists sparked a new round of major fires. As we huddled at home in front of our screens (if we were lucky and actually had electricity, which many people in California did not) we were introduced to murder hornets, the collective quest for toilet paper, hysteria and conspiracy theories about locked mailboxes, and, to top it all off, the emergent problem of an outsized feral "super-pig" population. It was not always possible to know when to laugh or cry. Alcohol purchases went through the roof. With gyms shut down, people sat, and sat, and sat, sometimes watching movies and eating, while frontline workers lost sleep caring for the sick or keeping vital supplies moving.

The seriousness and severity of the stress of the unknown and imposed by lockdown—particularly with respect to the psychological impact of being separated from human contact for an extended period of time—are hard to overstate. A June 2020 article in *The New York Times* noted the WHO's advisory concerning risks to mental health "wrought by anxiety and isolation," adding, "Digital platforms such as Crisis Text Line and Talkspace regularly reported spikes in activity through the spring. And more than half of American adults said the pandemic had worsened their mental health, according to a recent survey by the Kaiser Family Foundation."

There are any number of mental health conditions, particularly anxiety and depression, and behavioral disorders that can be made worse by stress. Certain populations—including caregivers, doctors, and medical workers—are especially vulnerable. Additionally, SARS-CoV-2 itself "might infect the brain or trigger immune responses that have additional adverse effects on brain function and mental health in patients," according to an article in *The Lancet*.

Challenges to individual mental health while attempting to protect one's physical health are one thing. Under severe pressure, the temptation to panic is all too real, especially at the onset of a crisis.

One of the reasons for the initial panic in early spring of 2020 was critical information from the experts was not disseminated early enough to reach the community before the crisis began. Rather than educating the public on who would be vulnerable, moral panic ensued to contain the virus. As the hospitals were rapidly overflowing and reports of bodies being stacked in refrigerated trucks began circulating, all people, regardless of age and risk factors, were convinced if they caught the virus they would die.

The rising panic was everywhere, including social media, where public health experts were warning of catastrophe.

Andy Slavitt, former administrator of the Centers for Medicare and Medicaid Services (CMS) under President Barack Obama, tweeted in early March:

> Currently experts expect over 1 million deaths in the U.S. since the virus was not contained & we cannot even test for it.

Bill Gates said in an interview with *The Economist* that millions more would die in this pandemic, and "freedom" hinders the disappointing U.S. response, while commending China by saying they "did a very good job of suppressing the virus" with the "typical, fairly authoritarian" approach, acknowledging "individual rights that were violated."

In contrast to other countries that have histories of prolonged collective exposure to severe social stressors such as government-sponsored repression, bombing campaigns, and domestic terrorism, the United States, on the whole, does not have experience in the kinds of severe, wide-scale challenges to mental health presented by a pandemic. It was not only the immediate crisis at hand people were concerned about, it was the fear of long-term damage, which has become more frustrating than terrifying.

People became frustrated as they were not able to congregate with family or friends, yet little information was provided as to why. Scientists have quickly learned that not all transmission events are created equally, and so-called "super-spreader events"— when a single person infects a large amount of other people—have played an enormous role in the transmission of the virus. In fact, research and models of transmission suggest approximately 10 to 20 percent of infected people are responsible for 80 percent of COVID-19 cases. This explains why a single indoor gathering can lead to a chain of infections that not only affects the attendees, but anyone else they may come in contact with in the following days. "In Arkansas, an infected pastor and his wife transmitted the virus to more than 30 attendees at church events over the course of a few days, leading to at least three deaths," according to *Scientific American*. "And these new cases spread to 26 more people, at least one of whom died." The CDC estimates about 50 percent of viral transmissions take place *before* the infected person has any symptoms. Since symptoms take an average of five to six days to show, there is an extended time frame for someone to be around other people, unknowing they are contagious, setting up for a potential super-spreading event.

Further information emerged and parents everywhere were breathing a sigh of relief that children were seemingly escaping unscathed from the virus; but the moment of solace was short-lived. Early reports of children developing a rare inflammatory disorder several weeks following a mild or asymptomatic infection prompted renewed terror and determination to protect the children. While the multisystem inflammatory syndrome affecting children made headlines every day for weeks, it quickly fell off the news waves as social unrest began to grow, leaving parents with little information on how the infection may harm their children.

As much as this book is about communicating information regarding the virus, it is also concerned with collective, social panic—especially of the sort that is inflamed by erratic information and the politicization of science.

The uncertainty of how long shutdowns should remain further incites panic and division. The fear of the unknown can be the greatest contributor to panic. Even when transmission levels were less than 1 percent in areas of the country, businesses were harshly restricted, forcing many to close. A study from China, and circulated by CNN, suggested that even when viral transmission is low, because of the risk of reintroduction, some level of restrictions should stay in effect until herd immunity is reached. Since the country was nowhere near natural herd immunity at the time of the study in April 2020 and a vaccine was only a pipe dream at that time, further panic arose, with people unsure when and how businesses would survive.

One half of the population began encouraging places stay closed until a vaccine became available, regardless of how much damage was done and how low viral transmission got, while the other side began advocating for individual freedoms—and were labeled as murderers.

Bill Gates said in the same interview referenced earlier that Trump supporters have brandished "freedom," complicating the U.S. response to the pandemic.

Indeed, the rhetoric and the divisive mood in the United States during the current pandemic have been prone to sharp extremes, strong emotions, and chaos and violence that incite anxiety. Starting literal and figurative fires, resorting to violence, blaming deaths on political opponents, and demonizing people who disagree with them seem to have become default responses to handling the fear and anger provoked by uncertainty.

If you have ever seen a sign saying "Keep Calm and Carry On" you may know that it originated in 1939, when the British government posted such signs to improve morale during the bombing campaign against the U.K. by the Nazis. This cultural ethos has no real equivalent in the United States.

SOCIAL UNREST

Although it was not until late summer of 2020 that the devastating fires—sparked by an incendiary device at a "gender reveal" party gone wrong—started to burn on the West Coast, the country was already a tinderbox in terms of social unrest by late spring.

In the early months of spring, President Trump had held multiple rallies during the presidential primary season with tens of thousands of people in attendance. After a pause during initial lockdowns, the events were resumed and immediately criticized on social media and among news media outlets calling them "death rallies."

@GAFollowers tweeted:

> How many will get sick and die? We know that some will.
> Maybe a lot. A crime in plain sight. Killing them softly with their
> rallies, with his words, killing them softly.

Following the Tulsa rally in the early summer, public health officials blamed the local rise in cases on the rallies, with several members of the Trump administration also testing positive after the gathering.

The scrutiny had some people scratching their heads, as mass gatherings had been occurring for over a month with much less fanfare.

Two months before the Tulsa rally, George Floyd, an unarmed Black man, died during the course of his arrest by Minneapolis police.

This horrifying event sparked massive protests, which quickly became violent, and resulted in loss of life and the destruction of businesses, not to mention outbreaks of domestic terrorism by professional activists. It was not always clear where the principled protests ended and the lawless violence began.

For months, all that Americans had heard was:

Be safe.

Science says to stay home.

Do your part to lessen the spread.

Then, all of a sudden, people were told it is fine—if not morally and politically obligatory—to go out in the streets and protest.

The understandable and in many cases commendable desire to engage in nonviolent protest against racism and social equality—which should be sharply distinguished from violent insurrectionist threats to safety and peace—came up against what we had been told were nonnegotiable, scientifically sanctioned dictates of public health. Yet it seemed those dictates were negotiable for some, but not for all.

In fact, prior to George Floyd's death, protests against lockdowns were occurring by mid-April; however, the media treated these protesters' rights quite differently, with *USA Today* saying, "Americans are blessed with rights of speech and assembly, but they are not given rights to put others at risk of falling ill and even dying."

Yet, a quote from an interview in *USA Today* surrounding the Black Lives Matter (BLM) protests portrays a different tone: "By protesting and reacting, that shows me that people still have a sense of humanity about them, and they believe . . . that their expression of how they feel and what they think can still have the desired effect."

When Democrats refused to rebuke the protesters for violating social-distancing guidelines, their message was that the measures being taken were superfluous if the cause was aligned with certain messages.

Its impressive how the Democrats went from the lockdown party to the burn-it-all-down party in less than 48 hours.

The reality is, any event bringing together thousands will have limited physical distancing for prolonged periods of time. The close sustained contact with shouting can cause respiratory droplets and aerosols to be emitted, potentially transmitting the virus. In both settings, rallies and protests, individuals travel distances, which can spread the virus from one community to another, a major factor in our country's lack of control of the pandemic.

People had been told that the dictates of their own consciences, particularly with respect to religious obligations and nonurgent health concerns, did not matter in the face of the supposedly ironclad, unambiguous demands of science that they stay home. Americans understood the potential consequences and therefore complied. Yet, when the dialogue changed abruptly to involve explicit assurances from public officials that large gatherings weren't really a problem as long as they were a certain type of protest, it was deeply frustrating.

Holes were poked into the previous recommendations to stay home behind a wall of protection, making a Swiss cheese effect of the "science"—full of holes and prone to spoil.

When challenged on the double standards that prevented people from gathering to pray together and kept restaurants and other businesses shuttered while allowing other people to gather and protest together, New York mayor Bill de Blasio remarked about the BLM protests that "anyone who thinks there's different rules for different people, again, is not trying very hard to see the reality. We're in the middle of a national crisis, a deep-seated national crisis. There is no comparison. I'm sorry, I do feel for the store owners. I really do."

In that simple statement, the new trajectory of the lockdowns became obvious. Had they truly wanted to *follow the science*, rather than the politics, in the fight against COVID-19, leaders might want to take a closer look at the dichotomy of allowing mass gatherings of protests while keeping smaller gatherings, and therefore less risk of viral transmission, restricted.

By early July churches, mosques, and other houses of worship were only open to 25 percent capacity. Meanwhile, de Blasio joined hundreds in the street to paint "Black Lives Matter" in front of Trump Tower on Fifth Avenue. As "science" forced playgrounds to be closed with locked chains restricting physical activity for children, the message was clear that political stunts that fall in line with popular opinion were okay.

That is not science.

It shouldn't have to be said that arbitrarily imposing one's own subjective notions of what constitutes a historical crisis upon one's fellow citizens is a violation of duty, as well as of the equal rights of all citizens.

One can wholeheartedly agree that racism is evil, dangerous, and a menace to civic and public health, while pointing out that it makes no scientific sense to say people can gather closely together in large groups for some causes but not for others.

Nothing could be more anti-scientific than pretending viruses respect moral and political principles, and that they won't infect people who are protesting in the service of a good cause.

Nonetheless, it quickly became evident that a two-tiered protocol was in order. If you were protesting, you could join all the large gatherings that you wanted. If, however, you wanted to go to church or hold a funeral for a loved one, you were out of luck. Americans were thus treated differently based not on science, but on a desire to promote some activities and prevent others without respect to the question of comparable medical risks posed by both.

The result of this incoherent approach by lawmakers and public health officials was whiplash, confusion, anger, revolt, and panic.

Add in neglect of medical care, increased alcohol and drug consumption, lack of exercise, social isolation, deaths of loved ones, unemployment, and financial stress, and you end up with a recipe for catastrophe. Once riots, fires, and pre-election uproar had been added to the mix, talk of violence and burning things down became common fare on social media. To be sure, there were countless examples of quiet heroism, but, on the whole, there was a common impression that the country was violently falling apart, with cities such as New York and Portland turning into a modern-day Gotham nightmare.

How did this happen? What were the mid-pandemic milestones? What could have been done differently?

Historically speaking, although outbreaks of dangerous viruses causing diseases such as Zika, Ebola, Middle East respiratory syndrome (MERS), and severe acute respiratory syndrome (SARS) have occurred in recent years, the effects have fortunately been negligible in the United States. In the case of the prior coronavirus outbreaks causing MERS and SARS, no deaths occurred in the U.S. Americans had a collective sense of being "immune" to pathogens that appeared in other nations. This probably contributed not only to complacency and an underappreciation of the true severity of the outbreak, but to difficulty in weathering the challenges of promoting well-being, especially those associated with public health initiatives.

I want to make several points here regarding our mindsets, our habits, and our shared ways of life. With respect to our mentalities and habits, we need to get help when we need it (easier to say than do during a pandemic, but still necessary) and take responsibility for controlling the aspects of our lives that we can control, such as exercising, eating right, and not drinking excessively or, of course, smoking.

With respect to our shared ways of life, we have not yet been able to find a middle ground between open-it-all-up mindsets and strict, stay-at-home lockdown orders that are culturally acceptable to enough people. An in-between compromise is ultimately what needs to happen in this country.

MIXED PUBLIC MESSAGING MAKING THINGS WORSE

One of the most striking aspects of the 1918 influenza pandemic was the scarcity of public health messages from the federal government—or other sources—until the death toll was already sky high. The guidance provided was scarce, and late in the day, so to

speak. There were no Centers for Disease Control and Prevention—
the agency specifically tasked with issuing such guidance.

Over the course of its history, the CDC has fallen prey to administrative bloat, misuse of funds, and loss of focus. Tellingly, a 2007
report from the late Senator Tom Coburn, MD, was titled "CDC
Off Center—A review of how an agency tasked with fighting and
preventing disease has spent hundreds of millions of tax dollars for
failed prevention efforts, international junkets, and lavish facilities,
but cannot demonstrate it is controlling disease."

While no single entity can be blamed for the earlier failure of
testing or even having the insight of the intricacies of the virus
itself, what about their messaging later on?

Perhaps the best we can say about the CDC's handling of public health messaging in the SARS-CoV-2 pandemic is that not all
of their many blunders were self-instigated. In one troubling instance, when the CDC posted information on its website saying
that asymptomatic people who had been exposed to the virus may
not need to be tested, this received a quick, well-deserved backlash,
as it was known by this point that identifying asymptomatic persons
is essential to lessen the transmission of the illness. They later had
to reverse course and encourage testing for such persons. But these
blunders and quick reversals occurred many times regarding various pieces of information and led to infighting across the nation.

No one who has followed the CDC's errors and mixed messaging was surprised to see a headline in late September announcing:
"CDC stumbles again, mistakenly posts 'draft' guidance about airborne Covid-19 spread."

One doctor was quoted in the same NBC News article as
saying, "The CDC is like a North Star in terms of guiding this
pandemic. . . . It's important that there is clear and concise communication so that everybody is on the same page. . . . Hopefully we
will get communication from the CDC to better understand why
they're walking back on what we already know to be factual."

If you are starting to get the impression that conflicting messages and squabbling between agencies and officials are hallmarks of any public health crisis, you are right. Such spats are not just inherent to democratic politics, however. A comparison between public health messaging in China and in the United States suggests that we are fortunate to even be allowed to get a glimpse into the amount of discord.

An article in *The Wall Street Journal* explored the public health messaging crisis at the Chinese equivalent of the CDC and found an agency in massive disarray. Through "interviews with Chinese doctors, officials and health experts; and foreign scientists and officials who have worked with China on disease control," they discovered a number of troubling problems.

First, "The China CDC missed early signals because hospitals didn't enter details in its real-time system, the technological core of its disease-surveillance efforts"; second, "The agency was out-flanked by local authorities intent on hiding bad news from China's leader and elevating Wuhan's national political status"; third, "National officials delayed the response by forbidding publication of any research on the virus without approval, and shared critical information with the outside world in early January only after unauthorized leaks forced their hand"; and, finally, "Financial and personnel problems hobbled the China CDC, which struggled to recruit and retain talented staff."

No one familiar with public health offices would pretend that the relationship between politicians, on the one hand, and officials and bureaucrats, on the other, is neatly harmonious. But the conflict, unfortunately, cannot be reduced to a cartoon-like opposition between lucid, transparent truth-seekers and shady connivers.

The reality is more prosaic: people juggle conflicting agendas and sometimes ignore information because it doesn't fit a narrative. This is not excusable, nor is it uncommon.

WHO CAN BE TRUSTED?

If public health agencies tasked specifically with getting the messaging right fail us, and politicians fail us as well, to whom should we turn?

Throughout the current pandemic, various people and groups have appointed themselves as watchdogs or whistleblowers.

Dr. Bandy Lee, a forensic psychiatrist at Yale, has blamed the spread of the pandemic on what she, without ever having met with President Trump, has diagnosed as his severe mental illness.

As the *Yale Daily News* reports, "The group that Lee leads, the World Mental Health Coalition, has released a 'Prescription for Survival,' which argues that the president is 'making a global pandemic worse.' " They assign his failure to his supposed mental illness.

The Prescription for Survival chides the American people for not heeding its previous announcements and judgments, and recommends that the public ignore the administration that it elected and listen instead to "the CDC and credentialed public health officials."

In other words, follow the science.

But when we look to the CDC, the WHO, and other organizations we have been told to follow we find, in addition to useful and important work, releases of misinformation, vulnerability to political influence, and ineptitude on various issues during the pandemic. When we turn to credentialed public health officials, we may find someone responsible or, on the other hand, we might find others enacting nonscientifically significant mandates.

To whom can we turn for trustworthy advice that is informed by consideration of the most recent scientific developments while encompassing the overall wellness of society?

Because of the politicization of science and resultant panic, this question has become much harder to answer. Not only has this left us in a state of chaos, but the challenge of whom we can trust to fix this is one of the reasons why I wrote this book.

The troubling truth is that we may be inclined to accept advice on the pandemic only from those whom we take to share at least some of our political and opinion commitments. This is a dangerous and disastrous tendency. While every profession has its bad apples, there are trustworthy doctors, public health officials, and yes, even some politicians on both sides of the political spectrum and in the middle, as well.

Ultimately, we need to get informed and stay informed, and to consider in addition to guidance from reliable sources what we can do as individuals.

The simple fact that the quest for treatments and a vaccine has become politicized is the most blatant example of the government and academic hacks influencing science. Most people who are distrusting, including the anti-vaxxers, are not anti-science, uneducated, ignorant individuals; rather, they have a deep distrust of the process and interests of large government, and want honest guidance.

While not all of us may have contributed to the hostile, fearful climate of panic afflicting our country, we can *all* play a role in combatting it. We can do this by setting good examples and, as simple as this may sound, treating others as we would like to be treated, which is actually very hard to do.

While we may get a quick rush of dopamine from saying harsh things on social media to someone we disagree with politically, does this really add to our individual and collective well-being?

When our nation's leaders are the epitome of discord, the national consciousness becomes transformed and the people's spirit is diminished. We have adapted new norms and beliefs based on the words from people we have trusted. Misplaced power within institutions has become questioned. An overall feeling of malfeasance has caused many to negate some of the most fundamental basics of protection during a public health crisis. The discord has caused some of the simplest theories to be rejected because of skepticism.

In this mess, we have lost rational dialogue and the ability to listen to scientists without assuming everyone has an agenda. We also have gotten to a point where shaming people, whether it's about masks or school preference, has become normalized if it doesn't agree with our philosophy. Moving forward, we need to transcend that. Let us look at the situation rationally, with empathy rather than fear and disdain driving each action, to put us back on the right path.

CHAPTER 3

FACE MASKS

Unmasking the Truth

A mask you ask? Optional I find!
Masks lend appeal of a mysterious kind.

—E.A. BUCCHIANERI, *PHANTOM PHANTASIA: POETRY FOR THE PHANTOM OF THE OPERA PHAN*

Historically speaking, many practices crucial to modern medicine, such as doctors washing hands in between patients and even wearing face masks, were derived from practicing clinicians who learned something through experience, not from a laboratory somewhere. Prior to the mid-19th century, hard though it may be to believe, many doctors had no research training at all. Today, all licensed doctors of medicine in the West have such education. Yet widespread confusion about the potential for disagreement between scientific research and the practice of medicine persists. And this discord, albeit common, is contributing to the panic over SARS-CoV-2.

It's natural to let fear and anger take over from time to time in our thoughts and feelings about certain matters, and to clutch at anything that promises relief.

Though, not all research findings will translate into best medical practice; in fact, most don't. What makes modern medicine "modern" to begin with is that the drugs, technologies, and innovations that it uses are the products of scientific progress built upon decades of trial and error.

As we place this in the context of COVID-19, when we hear about science and scientists, some uncertainty is always inevitable. Yet science is invoked as a source of absolutes, with many echoing the mantras that "science says" or "follow the science." Since people are desperate for clear answers, this is understandable, but also unfortunate.

This is not just a doomed error in understanding, however. It is a social problem—one that is fueling a public health crisis and costing human lives.

Misunderstanding what science can promise and deliver is what creates space for the politicization of science with respect to rhetoric. In that context, ignorance about how science works is dangerous but almost inevitable. Once ignorance fuels politicization, coloring basic research, governing its interpretation, and constraining clinical practice, it can turn fatal.

In the 21st century, mass hysteria and its sinister brother, conspiracy theory, can be just as dangerous as viruses, bacteria, and other pathogens. In previous centuries, contagion panics and conspiracy theories existed but were hard to transmit broadly and were contained locally. Now mass communications, newspapers, TV, and the internet make symptoms, warnings, and rumors globally available in seconds; it is possibly even more disruptive than acts of bioterrorism and envelopes of white powder.

The controversy over wearing face masks is a case in point identifying discord during COVID-19.

FACE MASKS

The prevailing word at the beginning of the pandemic was that unless you were sick, you didn't need to wear a face mask.

In truth, leading up to the introduction of SARS-CoV-2, much of the data was muddied regarding how effective public use of face masks was in lowering transmission of respiratory viruses, mainly because there wasn't an urgency to study it outside of China. Following the original SARS outbreak, a few studies emerged evaluating the effectiveness of the widespread use of reusable cloth masks. As we began the SARS-CoV-2 pandemic, it was these studies that people looked to for information. Yet, the results were interpreted differently. A U.S. study from 2010 suggested cloth masks had a filtration efficiency of 15 to 57 percent compared to the medical-grade N95 masks, concluding cloth masks have minimal effectiveness in protecting the wearer. While some may say that is clear evidence that they are ineffective, others may say they have *some* level of efficacy in reducing viral transmission. It is a glass-half-full versus glass-half-empty scenario. However, despite the limited existing data, there was *no* clinical research to inform public use and most existing policies offered no guidance on it.

Americans were explicitly told NOT to wear masks initially by not only U.S. infectious disease experts but also the World Health Organization. This was understandable, due to worries that frontline medical workers, who were most at risk, would not have enough masks if people began hoarding them. This was a very real fear, due in no small part to China having virtually cornered the world's supply of protective personal equipment (PPE) at a time when the rest of the world didn't know what was coming. In January alone, as *The New York Times* reported, China "bought up much of the rest of the world's supply. According to official data, China imported 56 million respirators and masks in the first week after the January lockdown."

Culturally, Americans, unlike citizens of countries where mask-wearing is common, weren't prepared to be told to wear masks. It was not something we were accustomed to. In countries such as China and Japan, masks serve as societal norms, functioning as the first line of defense against air pollution and pathogen transmission. However, most recent past pandemics did not result in generalized mask-wearing and the international ones that did, did not affect the United States.

Another important thing: COVID-19 has an abnormally large amount of presymptomatic and probably asymptomatic spread of the virus, which we didn't know at first. As this became obvious, the recommendations changed. By early April, many public health experts reached a consensus encouraging the public to wear a face mask to lower infection rates, even if some only offered a 15 percent reduction—the country was desperate.

As the WHO dragged their feet adopting the emerging evidence on viral transmission, the U.S. CDC recommended voluntary wearing of public face masks April 3; the WHO waited until June 5 before offering such recommendations.

Alas, the recommendation for Americans to start wearing face masks was met with twofold resistance, the questioning of data behind their effectiveness and asinine public behavior regarding them, both anti-science. What should have been a simple public health initiative turned into a mockery of science and ultimately polarized communities.

When people are being ridiculed for going to the beach or jogging alone in a park when not wearing a mask, and others are praised for their mask-wearing, even if doing so inappropriately or unnecessarily, people will feel like mask-wearing is nothing more than virtue-signaling nonsense. From this, the literary characters of the pandemic continued, with villains and anti-villains.

The tone of resistance to the face mask can be highlighted by various social media comments. For example, @kdmize44 October 2020 responded to a tweet encouraging mask-wearing:

> This seems like a lot of BS. We've never needed masks before. Political propaganda.

It certainly doesn't help the backlash when statements downplaying the seriousness of the pandemic and immature behaviors are made by policymakers and other people in the public eye.

Vanessa Hudgens, an actress well-known for portraying Gabriella

Montez in Disney Channel's High School Musical franchise, filmed a live video broadcast to her 38 million Instagram followers saying:

> Coronavirus is a bunch of bullshit. Like, I dunno, I think it'll last, like, a month?

But it isn't solely teenybopper, ill-informed celebrities misfeeding the public about the virus; public health officials were also making outlandish recommendations regarding preventive behaviors.

Canada's chief public health officer told people that "if you choose to engage in an in-person sexual encounter with someone outside of your household, consider wearing a mask that covers the nose and mouth." Sure, wearing a mask may lessen transmission of the virus, but let's be reasonable here: if two people are together enough to engage in such intimacy, a mask won't stop the spread of SARS-CoV-2.

While an extreme example, people also began wearing masks when unnecessary, the other end of the spectrum of not "following the science." Vox conducted a survey in late November 2020 asking people if they took their mask off while dining with a small group of people other than immediate household members. Seven percent of the respondents said they *never* remove their mask, even when they are eating and drinking. This response begs the question of how they are getting their food and beverage into their mouth without removing the mask that is covering their mouth. While the follow-up question wasn't asked or answered, one can surmise that the mask must be pushed aside briefly, possibly contaminating the hands or mouth at the same time. The thing is, masks may work when worn appropriately, but wearing them appropriately seems to be a challenge for some people.

Comedian Abbi Crutchfield tweeted in May:

> I just removed my mask to sneeze into my sleeve. Am I doing this right?

While that tweet seems on par for her stand-up routine as obvious satire, indeed, then-presidential candidate Joe Biden was cap-
tured on video lowering his mask to cough into his hand during a
campaign event.

Trump's default position was generally for individual accountability and individual outcomes, whereas Biden strongly voiced support
for generalized mask-wearing at all times, even saying a national
mask mandate would be a top priority, yet not clarifying what that
would mean for restaurants and other outdoor spaces.

Immediately, Trump and anyone who questioned the validity of
generalized mask-wearing were the anti-mask rogues and Biden and
those wearing masks, even when driving alone in their own personal cars, were the mask-wearing stars.

The ensuing clash propelled the investigation of whether widespread wearing of face masks would be a useful tool in combating
the novel virus to help lessen transmission rates.

However, science does not work absent the tolerance of uncertainty, because scientific research can't proceed without it. In actu-
ality, it is the presence of uncertainty that drives discovery, and it
is essentially a professional requirement for researchers to keep an
open mind. Research pursues to prove or disprove a question, not
necessarily establish a fact. These questions prompt experiments,
and experiments yield more or less certain findings—findings
which can be misconstrued.

"Because the issue has become so politicized, there's a real
risk—and it's already being used in this way—that studies like
this will be sort of cherry-picked and presented as conclusive evidence that masks are completely ineffective," Columbia University
virologist Angela Rasmussen told *The Washington Post*. And the
opposite is just as possible—that people will present masks as the
end-all-be-all to save the country. Still, if you were to examine
public opinion, there clearly appears to be no room for anywhere
in between the two extremes, both claiming to *follow the science*.
So who is right?

THE SCIENCE

The primary reason to wear a face mask is to protect others from asymptomatic and presymptomatic transmission, but growing evidence is showing a level of protection for the wearer as well. While wearing a mask may not unequivocally prevent someone from contracting the virus, it can also decrease the viral load, leading to less severe symptoms.

Since most face mask research has been conducted on influenza viruses, data was lacking at the beginning of the pandemic, so researchers worked quickly to determine if face masks would be a tool against SARS-CoV-2.

A variety of face masks ranging from a simple homemade cloth mask to ventilated respirators have all played a role in the current COVID-19 pandemic.

The sharp increase in demand for medical face masks resulted in an acute shortage as the country was dependent on a global supply chain. In order to help the shortage, researchers were hastily working to explore whether alternative coverings such as homemade cloths masks, gaiters, and others that are readily available and affordable would work.

By mid-August, *The Wall Street Journal* reported the existence of "growing evidence that facial coverings help prevent transmission— even if an infected wearer is in close contact with others."

It cited recent studies, including one in *Physics of Fluids*, which showed that "Well-fitted homemade masks with multiple layers of quilting fabric, and off-the-shelf cone style masks, proved to be the most effective in reducing droplet dispersal. These masks were able to curtail the speed and range of the respiratory jets significantly, albeit with some leakage through the mask material and from small gaps along the edges."

A study out of Singapore published in September 2020 also evaluated the ability of various face masks to stop SARS-CoV-2 transmission. The results showed multilayer cotton and surgical masks significantly reduced the number of particles expelled, with a reduction of 86.4 percent and 99.9 percent, respectively. However, the study revealed that some mask alternatives, such as single-layer coverings like neck gaiters and bandanas, offered little protection against infection, similar to prior studies on SARS.

Even anecdotal evidence has shown that wearing masks can be effective at preventing spread of the virus. Paul Best of Fox News reported, "For instance, two hairstylists in Missouri saw 140 clients earlier this summer while infected with COVID-19, but none of the clients ended up contracting the disease, which health officials attributed to the workers wearing masks."

The University of Washington's Institute for Health Metrics and Evaluation began tracking COVID-19 cases, taking into account mobility data, testing, mask use, population density, air pollution, altitude, annual pneumonia death rate, smoking, and self-reported contacts. After assessing the covariates and reported rate of mask use, it concluded "mask use results in up to 50% reduction in transmission of COVID-19."

MASKS MANDATES

By April, it was apparent that, as the authors of an article in the *American Journal of Tropical Medicine and Hygiene* noted, "resistance to mass masking seems inconsistent with our knowledge of the rate of asymptomatic infections and the risk of transmission from these individuals," adding that "laboratory data support both surgical and cloth masks," despite the need for further inquiry into cloth masks.

The political debate concerning mask mandates was heating up as many private business owners and governors installed such mandates in their areas of control. To further add to the conversation, Joe Biden recommended that the federal government—as distinguished from state and local governments—mandate generalized public mask wearing at *all* times.

Yet even as the scientific evidence continued to grow showing that masks represented a viable way of reducing transmission because of the high proportion of asymptomatic and presymptomatic transmission, there was a lack of evidence of the magnitude of such effects, especially at a population level.

By late October, 59 percent of polled voters expressed support for a national mask mandate in a *New York Times*/Siena College poll, down from 67 percent in September.

To date, a majority of U.S. states have enacted some type of mask mandate, but one of the biggest uproars has been from people on various platforms insisting that cases went up after mask mandates were in place, questioning the benefit.

@lindabirdd tweeted:

> I'm in Minnesota. We have a mask mandate and everywhere I go the majority of people are properly wearing a mask. Minnesota positive case have done nothing but go up since it started. I'll never be convinced simple cloth or surgical masks can prevent the virus spread.

Following a comment advising the wearing of masks to lessen community transmission, Jane Hughes, a medical doctor and self-reported conservative, tweeted:

> Look at California new cases and look when masks were mandated . . . cases continued to climb, exponentially. Rethink your position.

Numerous posts across all social media platforms put forth graphs showing when mask mandates were instituted followed by a rise in cases, with some even suggesting mask mandates may actually spread COVID-19.

As many states passed mandates while their neighboring states were exploding with cases, it was inevitable for there to be some rise in transmission since interstate travel was never halted. And it really takes two to four weeks before any public health strategies or major events will show up in the data.

So if we look to the data, specifically in Minnesota to address @lindabirdd's tweet, roughly three weeks following when the indoor mask mandate went into effect, the 14-day rolling average of daily confirmed cases declined 14 percent.

Now let's do California. In mid-June, Governor Gavin Newsom issued a mandate for people to wear a face mask when in public areas, yet cases continued to rise. The state is so big—the population of California is larger than that of Canada—and there's a lot of different things going on in different places. The *Los Angeles Times* performed a survey reporting only 42 percent of the people observed were wearing masks correctly, with 10 percent wearing them incorrectly and 47 percent not wearing masks at all, calling it a "mask rebellion." So is it really a surprise that cases went up when over half of the population was not wearing masks as recommended? By the end of the fall, California surpassed a million cases, leading to more restrictive mitigation efforts.

But people rejecting masks was not the sole reason California became the nation's epicenter of the pandemic; there were many contributing factors, including emerging, more infectious viral variants as well as other factors, much of which are unique to California's geographical location and demographics.

Throughout the state, while Latinos make up 39 percent of the population, they make up the largest share of COVID-19 cases (56 percent) and deaths (42 percent), according to data from the California Department of Public Health. Not only are outbreaks occurring throughout the Latino community, but according to contact tracing and epidemiological studies, much of it is within low-income communities living in crowded housing, often where people are essential workers unable to work remotely, yet who cannot afford to call in sick. Language, immigration status, and financial issues can complicate efforts to convince them to be tested and isolate themselves for extended periods. Also, with hospitalizations in California increasing over 90 percent during the holiday season, part of what is driving some of this overflow is the influx of positive patients from Mexico. State officials report that hundreds of thousands living in neighboring Baja are crossing back in search of superior health care.

Not to mention, over 4,000 prisoners tested positive in California prison systems, many requiring transfer to local hospitals. Lastly, the homelessness epidemic, with over 150,000 Americans living on the streets of California, is another major risk factor for harboring SARS-CoV-2.

California went into the pandemic in a precarious position, with the über-wealthy living in their designated zip codes, the younger generations still going out to hit the bars and beaches, and then the vulnerable who were left as sitting ducks with little available funding as the state continuously nears bankruptcy. Had the state been more fiscally conservative in the past, they might have had the funding to provide more support to break language and cultural barriers to educate residents on ways, specifically mask-wearing, to lessen the spread.

Far away from the Pacific with an entirely different subset of demographics, North Dakota had the lowest mask-wearing rate in the country by October, according to survey data, also having the highest per capita COVID-19 infection rate of any state in the country, according to the CDC. While Republican governor Doug Burgum refused to implement a mandate for the public to wear masks, they found themselves in such a situation that the governor told COVID-positive health care workers to stay on the job as they were suffering a staff shortage from frontline medical workers falling ill from COVID-19. Shortly after this despairing move, the governor conceded and implemented a mask mandate in mid-November, when the state was reporting fewer than 15 available ICU beds in the state, as cases were continuing to rise.

Yet, North Dakota was not the only state without a mask policy; actually, eight of the ten states with the highest new cases per capita during the winter holiday months did not have a widespread mask mandate.

Because of this obvious trend, research began to shift from the focused efficacy of a mask to prevent viral transmission to the effectiveness of mask-wearing on a population level. If policymakers were going to force people to wear masks or even recommend it, they had better be able to back up their actions with indisputable science to prevent further "mask rebellion."

A study performed at the University of Utah demonstrated that statewide mask mandates were able to not only reduce the spread of SARS-CoV-2 but also help businesses during the concomitant economic crisis. The researchers noted that not only do COVID-19 cases decrease after mask orders are put in place, but consumer mobility and spending increase after mask mandates are enacted. While they noted statewide mask mandates seemed to be more effective than county-level requirements, county-level trends evaluated by the CDC suggest even countywide mandates appear to have contributed to the mitigation of viral transmission in the specific counties.

Kansas was a state that held out on declaring a statewide mandate and rather implemented 24 county mandates in the counties with considerably higher infection rates. Although those counties were starting at a disadvantage, the data showed the implementation of mask mandates reversed the increasing trend in COVID-19 incidence, whereas counties that did not have mask mandates continued to experience increasing cases.

Another analysis from Vanderbilt University School of Medicine highlighted how Tennessee COVID-19 hospitalizations rose at a much lower rate in areas that had mask mandates than in those that did not. Studies are consistently showing declines in COVID-19 cases observed in another 15 states and the District of Columbia, which mandated masks, compared with states that did not have mask mandates. The *Health Affairs* article evaluating the trend noted that mandates led to a slowdown in daily COVID-19 growth rate, which became more apparent over time as there is a one-to-three-week lag in preventative measures and new cases being reported. Other studies found that countries with preexisting cultural norms or government policies promoting mask-wearing before COVID had lower death rates overall.

In one simulation, researchers predicted that had 80 percent of the population initially been told to wear masks, this may have done more to reduce COVID-19 spread than the subsequent lockdown measures that followed. Yet, our health officials told us not to wear masks—a major blunder that not only eroded confidence in their effectiveness but also led to lives lost and economic ruin for many.

While many studies have come forward showing the benefit of mask-wearing, all it took was a pdf of an antiquated irrelevant study or a single flawed contemporary study to thrust the legitimacy of mask-wearing back into the limelight.

THE DANISH STUDY

Referring to a tweet I sent out saying "masks aren't fool proof, but they do lessen transmission when worn appropriately," @TriBeCaDad responded,

> But there's a new Dutch study that contradicts what you just said

In mid-November a study from Denmark, named DANMASK-19 (Danish Study to Assess Face Masks for the Protection Against COVID-19 Infection), was published in the *Annals of Internal Medicine* that made headlines and began trending on social media.

The reason the study grabbed attention was because they reported *no statistically significant difference* between infection rates among a group of people who wore face masks and a group of people who did not wear them. However, like most clinical research, a single line hardly explains the study.

The researchers tabulated how many cases of COVID-19 there were into two groups, with 42 cases in the group who wore face masks and 53 infections in the other group. So while there was a 26 percent increased risk of getting COVID-19 in the group who didn't wear masks, because of the small infection numbers and not enough cases to power the study, it was deemed not statistically significant.

However, when you read through the methods and additional information outside of the paper's abstract, it details how only 46 percent of the people in the face mask–wearing group actually reported wearing them as instructed (over the nose and mouth while outside of the home). They did not specify what it meant for the other groups that reported wearing them "predominately as recommended" and "not as recommended." They also did not specify whether people who got COVID-19 reportedly wore the mask as recommended or not.

So, if we play with the numbers and factor in the people who did not wear a mask appropriately, adding them to the group that didn't wear a mask, then it's plausible there is up to a 57 percent increased risk of getting COVID-19 if not wearing a mask or not wearing one appropriately—which falls in line with other contemporary data. While the criticism of the study is not limited to this, another factor that has drawn analysis is that it used mostly antibody tests to determine infection, one with a reported 2.5 percent false positive rate. Since less than 2 percent of the people in the study got COVID, you can't look for a 2 percent effect with a test that has a 2.5 percent false positive. That would indicate over half of the positive cases in this study were potentially false positives.

Ultimately, there were many factors in this study that may have raised concern in the review process and should have been addressed prior to publication. While the anti-mask group clamored at the lack of statistical significance, even the lead author of the study commented during an interview that the research was being taken out of context and that he believed the data showed there was effectiveness in wearing face masks. In fact, in the conclusion of the study (for those who read the entire thing), the authors wrote, "Although no statistically significant difference in SARS-CoV-2 incidence was observed, the 95% CIs are compatible with a possible 46% reduction to 23% increase in infection among mask wearers."

Yet, the mixed messages confuse people, and confusion can be unnerving in times of uncertainty and turmoil.

Pending consistent herd immunity status, SARS-CoV-2 is here to stay. Even with a vaccine, the virus will likely become endemic to our society, with many variants, meaning rather than our having "flu season" every year, it may be "flu and COVID season." We can and do complain about it but we have to dance with it, and that means adopting measures to lower the transmission of the virus as more people gain natural and vaccine-induced immunity.

While it is true that mask mandates will certainly not end the pandemic alone, there isn't much proof of much else, certainly not enough to counter the strong argument backed by scientific evidence showing lessened transmission with mask-wearing when appropriate.

It is important to reiterate that rarely will there ever be universal consensus on anything scientific. Anyone can do a Google search to find a research study saying what they want it to say; it doesn't make them right and the other people wrong. However, if many of the negative claims about mask-wearing were true, we would have seen major liability issues of health care workers dropping like flies, as we have been wearing the most robust face masks for extended periods of time for decades.

Scientists cannot spend their days focused on dispelling irrational (or rational but incorrect) mask concerns. Anyone can make any claim about masks. The quest to disprove them is futile.

While we can't argue people out of their beliefs, we can perhaps move their thinking adjacent to their views through clear, concise, and transparent information regarding even the possibility of a benefit to mask-wearing.

Wearing a mask isn't 100 percent foolproof, and anyone who says differently is lying. However, lessening the risk of viral transmission is all that is needed, until the vulnerable are protected with long-term immunity.

One reason that many people avoid cigarette smoking is to prevent cancer. But not smoking doesn't guarantee that one will never get cancer. Rather, we avoid certain behaviors, like tobacco use, not for an absolute certainty, but to reduce the likelihood of negative outcomes. Liken this to wearing a seat belt—it doesn't guarantee you will survive the car crash, but it certainly reduces the risk of dying.

The moment public health officials were aware of sustained spread within the United States given the highly transmissible nature of the virus, the message of risk reduction by mask-wearing should have been hammered into the American people and maybe we would have avoided much of the controversy and the need for mandates.

We didn't need a mandate. We didn't need to be forced to stay home. We needed transparent education and advice on the potential benefit of such actions, even if the science was unclear. The concept of mask-wearing to lessen the spread is not too complex for people to understand, it has just been misconstrued. Telling people to try something that *may* help is too mundane and less emotionally satisfying than debating it out among perceived villains and heroes. Unfortunately, delaying preventive measures, even if wholly unproven, has penalties.

CHAPTER 4

RESEARCH UNDER PRESSURE

Polarization Closes Minds and Hinders Progress

It is a capital mistake to theorize before one has data. Insensibly, one begins to twist facts to suit theories, instead of theories to suit facts.

—SHERLOCK HOLMES

The necessity of refusing to lie to oneself and others—of refusing to pretend that certainty exists when it does not—is even more profound for people who have been trained in the sciences. Indeed, in the context of learning, it is unethical to pretend that a question is settled (and thus, beyond questioning) when it has not been. As physicist Richard Feynman remarked:

It is imperative in science to doubt; it is absolutely necessary, for progress in science, to have uncertainty as a fundamental part of your inner nature. To make progress in understanding, we must remain modest and allow that we do not know. . . . You investigate for curiosity, because it is *unknown*, not because you know the answer. And as you develop more information in the sciences, it is not that you are finding out the truth, but that you are finding out that this or that is more or less likely.

Admittedly, this sort of modesty is hard to come by in the midst of a pandemic, as loved ones die alone in hospitals, and people's jobs and basic well-being crumble into ruin. Given the extent to which we turn to science for clear, unambiguous answers and guidance, it makes sense that we might be inclined to lash out at anyone and everyone who stands in its way.

Yet, we are clamoring for the quick fix, the saving grace, anything to pull us out of this crisis. But our desperation should not persuade us to accept something that may not be wholly reliable, especially as financial incentives often result in expensive solutions. In fact, Big Pharma tends to wield much of its financial support and power from Big Government, particularly in times of crisis.

The relationship between the two entities began a century ago, around 1920, marked by the discovery and subsequent distribution of penicillin and insulin. Demands for pain-relieving medications and more antibiotics intensified during World War II, so the government collaborated with various international drug companies to mass-produce the remedies. The first-time trial of this sort of alliance opened the door for further collaboration between private industry and the federal government.

The 1976 campaign to vaccinate "every man, woman, and child" during a swine flu outbreak is still talked about today as one of the greatest failures from government and industry alliance. Dreading another deadly flu pandemic, under President Gerald Ford, a mass vaccination campaign was initiated. In order to get drug companies to speedily manufacture the vaccine, the government declared the drug companies would not be liable if there were any bad reactions to the vaccines.

This is somewhat reminiscent of New York governor Andrew Cuomo removing liability from nursing homes and hospitals following the institution of his nursing home order. When you take away potential culpability of actions, less care may be taken to assure checks and balances have been confirmed.

Following a rise in a rare neurological disorder called Guillain-Barré syndrome and at least 25 deaths due to mass vaccinations, the swine flu vaccination campaign of 1976 was suspended. By then, 45 million Americans had already been injected. Meanwhile, the feared crisis never evolved into a pandemic, but the credibility of the government and pharmaceutical alliance was stained.

Today, the pharmaceutical industry contributes heavily to many federal programs, including the U.S. Food and Drug Administration (FDA), not to mention millions of dollars being paid for lobbying. Medical journals, academic health care systems, and researchers across the world all accept money from the pharmaceutical industry for the purpose of scientific discovery and implementation.

In reality, the pharmaceutical industry reveals a disturbing truth: while they offer potentially life-saving benefits, they remain one of the least trusted entities—maybe only second to the skepticism surrounding Big Government. When you add the two bodies together, cynicism is amplified.

They certainly don't make it easy for us to trust the benevolence behind federal and industry collaboration when glaring conflicts of interests are present in appointing federal leaders. For example, in respect to COVID-19, the appointment of former pharma executive Moncef Slaoui to lead the White House's initiative Operation Warp Speed (OWS) left many people speechless. OWS, now a household name but a bold and unknown endeavor at the beginning of the crisis, provided crucial funding toward research, development, and manufacturing of many vaccine candidates. Slaoui has decades of experience in immunology, ample experience overseeing vaccine production, and intimate knowledge of the pharmaceutical industry and FDA process, all of which are crucial to the success of OWS. However, many questioned how much this person stood to gain from the expensive solutions produced by the mass effort. After criticism, he sold off $12.4 million worth of stock in Moderna (one of the leading vaccine contenders backed by OWS) but kept his shares in a biotech company (Lonza Group) that was contracted with Moderna to manufacture its vaccine. He also chose not to sell his stock in GlaxoSmithKline, estimated to be worth $10 million, another company backed by OWS to produce a vaccine. While he may be the most qualified person for the job, the many ways he stands to financially gain from the efforts cast suspicion on the process.

Drug companies, as well as anything related to health care delivery, have a powerful hold over people, as the ability to live a healthy life can seemingly depend on these companies' ability to produce the solution. Ultimately, people should be skeptical of Big Pharma, Big Government, and any answer put forward that is based on extremely expensive solutions.

For the current pandemic, the combination of personal responsibility and innovation are doing what we wanted: not just flattening the curve, but ultimately saving lives. From spring through the end of 2020, analyses had shown mortality rates of hospitalized patients in the United States having dropped from 11.4 percent to 3.7 percent, with the average length of stay in the hospitals declining from 10.5 days in March to less than five days in the fall months. Other studies, including data from the American Hospital Association, further suggest that the number of fatalities per infection fell by 20 percent during the course of the year, before vaccines became available.

As we will discuss further in this chapter, none of the treatments produced by the Goliath drug companies have proven to be "magic bullets" resulting in monumental improvement in survivability—rather, methods with less pomp and circumstance contributed more to the result.

It's important to examine the controversy that formed in the quest for treatments that ultimately led to saving lives. We must also consider how it bears upon larger questions of how the politicization of science not only hinders popular perceptions of truth but can alter the work of scientists themselves.

In order to carry out its work, experimental science needs political protection, financial support, and regulation with respect to living subjects. Crucially, it also needs independence. The balance between these goals must be continually worked out.

One major reason for optimism about the U.S. health care system is that it values private innovation, while discouraging intellectual theft. Such potential has started to be tapped on a national scale during the SARS-CoV-2 cataclysm. We have varying levels of invention in an all-hands effort to drive drug and vaccine trials in the face of vast political headwinds.

There have been some worrisome failures of responsibility in the rush to produce results. The advance of science, however, doesn't depend on the elimination of messiness, haste, and error but rather on reducing their frequency and their consequences.

Ironically, scientists themselves are more comfortable with the messy nature of science than are the public and especially journalists, particularly the ones who cherry-pick favorite scientists and then announce that their judgments are simply what "science says" rather than engaging a range of perspectives among experts. The narrative of a clear-cut partisan battle between ignorant foes of science and noble champions of it makes the media's job much easier.

Any event or piece of data in the pandemic can be treated as a crisis and used as evidence to support one candidate for office or indict another. Many members of the media know that, to borrow a trite cliché from the history of newspaper journalism, "if it bleeds, it leads." But this does not explain why some victims' stories are sensationalized, and others ignored.

This is a time of great trial for the press, but also one of great opportunity. The mass media can act not only as a clearinghouse for accurate, sober information and a source of intelligent, careful analysis, but also as a forum for thoughtful ideas about action.

The real story doesn't feature a dramatic battle between evil villains who don't care about human lives fighting noble heroes untainted by self-interest, but rather, flawed human beings trying to achieve results in the face of huge, chronically defective regulatory and governmental systems that would surely benefit from targeted reforms. All the while, media outlets and crisis entrepreneurs sell inflammatory narratives, and responsible journalists try to combat the myths. For their part, scientists have to grapple with both the heroic and non-heroic dimensions of science, and work hard to defend the distinction between science and politics, which cynics might dismiss as an illusion foisted on us by those in power.

Up until this point, the country depended on antiquated means to save lives as the race for treatments and vaccines was underway. As the months went by, progress was being made, yet the political interference became profound.

NATURAL REMEDIES

Drinking tea. Staying warm. Taking herbal mixtures full of mint, turmeric, honeysuckle, forsythia, or licorice or some combination thereof. Could an effective treatment for SARS-CoV-2 really lie in such a seemingly simple (and inexpensive) approach?

When the novel coronavirus first arose in Wuhan, no one familiar with the contemporary history of China was surprised that the government immediately started pushing Traditional Chinese Medicine (TCM) as a remedy for it. Chairman Xi Jinping, as is widely known, promotes TCM as a national cultural treasure that China wants to share with the world.

Yu Yanhong, the deputy head of the National Administration of Traditional Chinese Medicine, remarked back in March 2020, "We are willing to share the 'Chinese experience' and 'Chinese solution' of treating COVID-19, and let more countries get to know Chinese medicine, understand Chinese medicine, and use Chinese medicine."

Although the efficacies of some TCM remedies for SARS-CoV-2 continue to be tested, most researchers say the TCM trials have not been rigorously designed and are unlikely to produce reliable results. Due to Chinese censorship, criticism of TCM is somewhat muted, so without the criticism of the methods, the one-sided promotion of its "benefit" across media platforms goes undisputed.

Unproven natural remedies for the new disease weren't restricted to only China. Other countries, like Madagascar, had their own "cure" based on observed effects in a handful of people who took the solution. Madagascar president Andry Rajoelina openly hawked an herbal drink made from the artemisia plant—one he called "Covid-Organics"—and claimed that it could cure people with COVID-19. Yet he refused to release the ingredients of the solution for scientists to study and evaluate, fearing the recipe might be stolen.

To be fair, there is diminutive convincing evidence for *any* nontraditional medicine, not just those promoted by the Chinese and Malagasies. While the natural and various herbal preparations that line the shelves of American pharmacies and health-food stores generate millions, if not billions, of dollars every year, there is little concrete evidence of benefit to much of them.

However, where COVID-19 is concerned, there have been a few particular nutrients that garnered attention throughout the world as the pandemic raged on, specifically vitamin D. This vitamin was not only sought as a treatment for the illness, but became the center of government conspiracy theories.

Let me explain.

VITAMIN D

The 2002 outbreak of SARS created unprecedented levels of demand in the Chinese vitamin industry. The demand was so great that supplies of vitamin C, in particular, were severely depleted globally. The Chinese market for vitamins and supplements underwent a major expansion from that point forward.

In the pre-COVID era, there was question as to whether there is a direct link between the seasonality of influenza and vitamin D deficiency from decreased sun exposure. Since the prevalence of the viral infections may be higher in colder months from people congregating indoors, that same behavior may also lessen the amount of vitamin D in one's system.

Vitamin D is synthesized by our body as sunlight is absorbed through our skin. The vitamin is essential for several reasons, including maintaining healthy bones and teeth and preventing various diseases, such as diabetes and certain cancers. Additionally, as it comes into context during the current pandemic, it supports the immune system and lung function. This has been reinforced from years of data, including a 2018 review of existing research suggesting vitamin D has a protective effect against the influenza virus.

In the present case of SARS-CoV-2, both within China and beyond, there has been considerable interest in the general relationship between vitamin D and its ability to prevent and treat symptoms of COVID-19.

By May, after the virus had been circulating the globe for several months, a report in the *BMJ* made a case for a prudent blend of optimism and caution with respect to vitamin D and SARS-CoV-2:

> As a key micronutrient, vitamin D should be given particular focus—not as a "magic bullet" to beat COVID-19, as the scientific evidence base is severely lacking at this time—but rather as part of a healthy lifestyle strategy to ensure that populations are nutritionally in the best possible place.

Unfortunately, a direct consequence of increasing sun protection to lessen skin cancer risk has resulted in decreasing levels of vitamin D in developed countries for years. Studies have shown a lack of sun exposure from sunscreen, clothing cover-ups, and sun avoidance has resulted in about half of the elderly population having some level of vitamin D deficiency. This deficiency reduces the body's immune response and can increase the risk of infection.

By mid-September, researchers at Boston University School of Medicine analyzed data from 235 people who were hospitalized with

COVID-19 and echoed what was already suspected. They found patients older than age 40 were over half as likely to die from COVID if they did not have sufficient levels of vitamin D in their body.

Of further concern regarding our decreasing vitamin D levels, during the pandemic people are being told they can't spend time at the beach, play on playgrounds, or participate in group sports, and to isolate or quarantine indoors. The overall result of these measures is depriving people of sunlight and potentially lessening vitamin D absorption. Also, when people are spending time outdoors now, unless they are alone, a face mask covers over half the surface area of the face. As such, people have begun to theorize the government is intending harm upon us. An example from Twitter:

@brad_kemp45
For humans, the main source of VitD is its synthesis in the skin under the influence of solar ultraviolet radiation. And yet our LAW prohibits exposure of human bodies to sunshine in any public place. Tyranny/Prudery, misanthropy causes HARM and KILLS PEOPLE.

@njman421 remarked, referencing New Jersey governor Phil Murphy:

Get vitamin D while you can because Phil Murphy will steal your sunshine.

@lessshoe commented:

Quarantine nazi's are stopping us from getting vitamin D.

While some may theorize the government is intentionally lowering our vitamin D levels, there is little evidence to entertain that. Also, even a little critical thinking would show that rendering an entire population vulnerable to an illness wouldn't be good for policymakers who bank on being reelected and depend on working Americans' taxpaying dollars to fund their endeavors. If the reverse were true and the official advice was for everyone to take vitamin D as a preventive measure for COVID-19 and the government were to ship out a bottle to every American household, the same people accusing the government of intentionally decreasing vitamin D would probably be the same who refuse the charity shipment of the vitamin on the account the government was trying to control or poison them.

Undoubtedly vitamin D is proving to be essential for overall wellness and lessened severity of COVID-19. While our increased sunscreen use, staying inside, and wearing face coverings may decrease vitamin D levels, it is important to point out how easily people are able to get sufficient vitamin D through diet, limited sun exposure, and physician-prescribed supplements, if necessary. According to the Vitamin D Council, a fair-skinned person only needs to be outside for 15 minutes with some skin exposure to absorb ample rays for synthesizing vitamin D. The same absorption can take a couple of hours for people with darker skin, but the more exposed skin, the faster vitamin D can be made from the sun's rays. Certain people have a lower ability to make vitamin D naturally, including the obese, elderly, and those with liver and kidney disease. Coincidentally, these are the populations that also are disproportionately vulnerable to COVID-19.

Bottom line, if the mask-wearing is causing angst about lessening vitamin D levels, wear short sleeves and walk around the neighborhood twice a day—that will make up for the little real estate being covered up on the face.

As with every other proposed remedy currently available, there is no cause for unimpeachable confidence that higher-than-normal levels of vitamin D is a game changer in the treatment of COVID-19. No one should go out and consume vast quantities of it or, alternatively, dismiss it as irrelevant—as in the majority of life's circumstances, moderation is key. And in most cases, naturally derived, adequate levels from a healthy lifestyle *before* a person gets sick has greater benefit than artificial supplementation after the fact. Preventative health and wellness are the strongest tools we have against not only COVID-19, but most of our leading causes of death.

REMDESIVIR

Remdesivir is an antiviral medication that has become quite famous throughout the course of the pandemic. Prior to the discovery of SARS-CoV-2, it was a drug being researched for its ability to interfere with viral replication in the early stage of infection. While the medication garnered some enthusiasm pre-COVID as it showed decreased viral replication in *in vitro* (test tube) and animal *in vivo* studies against the coronaviruses that cause MERS and SARS, it had yet to be proven in human studies. Researchers and doctors were frantically looking for an existing treatment as hospitals were overflowing with critically ill COVID-19 patients in the early spring, so remdesivir began being used throughout the country under a compassionate use program as a possible remedy.

Early on, given the pressure to find therapies for COVID-19, small clinical trials without control groups were popping up all over the world with mixed results, but none showed a significant clinical benefit of the drug.

In April 2020, Dr. Fauci announced that a clinical trial supported by the U.S. National Institute of Allergy and Infectious Diseases (NIAID) with more than 1,000 people showed that those who were hospitalized taking remdesivir recovered in 11 days on average, compared with 15 days for those who received a placebo. This was the first piece of encouraging news the medical community had received indicating a possible way to shorten recovery time of hospitalized patients.

"Although a 31% improvement doesn't seem like a knockout

100%, it is a very important proof of concept," Fauci said. "What it has proven is that a drug can block this virus."

The data to which Dr. Fauci was referring were published in *The New England Journal of Medicine* the following month, in which the finding that "Remdesivir was superior to placebo in shortening the time to recovery in adults hospitalized with Covid-19 and evidence of lower respiratory tract infection" was reported. This was a randomized, double-blind, placebo-controlled trial, just the sort recognized to be the gold standard in assessing the efficacy of treatments.

Fauci further reminisced, as reported by *Nature*, that the remdesivir data "reminded him of the discovery in the 1980s that the drug AZT helped to combat HIV. The first randomized, controlled clinical trial [of AZT] showed only a modest improvement, but researchers continued to build on that success, eventually developing highly effective therapies," with people living longer with HIV than many other diseases.

Although being used by other pathways, by October remdesivir became the first medication given clearance by the FDA in the treatment of COVID-19.

The medication is administered via IV and requires six to eleven infusions for the treatment course. The company itself recommends only patients in a hospital setting should use remdesivir. In addition to the cost of administering it, the company put a hefty $3,120 price tag on it for insured patients in the United States. As more people began utilizing the medication, the drug brought in $873 million in sales the first full quarter it was on the market.

It needed to catch up, as the company reported spending $1 billion in research, development, and manufacturing while the Center for Integration of Science and Industry determined that between studying remdesivir's structure and target, the NIH also invested as much as $6.5 billion from 2000 to 2019.

For most, the existing contempt toward Big Pharma profiteering was quickly eroded by the hope that they could halt the virus and return life to normal.

While remdesivir may not be the miracle cure everyone is searching for, the fact that it was shown in multiple studies to shorten time to recovery gave enough hope that it would lessen the burden on the hospitals and continue additional scientific pathways to discover new medications and treatments.

However, as reported by Keith Speights at *The Motley Fool*, "Gilead's huge Q3 sales for remdesivir were made before the results from the largest clinical study evaluating the drug in treating COVID-19 patients were released. That's probably a good thing for the company."

The World Health Organization published interim data from their Solidarity Trial, which included more than 11,000 people across 30 countries evaluating medications (including remdesivir) as potential treatments of COVID-19. Not only did the medication not reduce death in the study, but the data also indicated remdesivir didn't influence the duration of hospitalizations, as previously reported.

As such, the WHO formally recommended that physicians not use the medication for COVID-19. While the WHO panel acknowledged that the collective evidence so far does not prove remdesivir "has no benefit," they discussed given the possibility of harm (adverse effects documented in 50 to 74 percent of people taking the medication), as well as the high cost and resources needed to administer the drug, the lack of clear evidence of benefit did not outweigh the risk.

However, given that Dr. Fauci publicly recognized the efficacy of remdesivir, the media depicted it as the "good" or hope-inducing drug, so the process pressed on. Since the medication requires hospitalization to administer, anecdotally, people were reporting being hospitalized only to receive the drug, with mixed results as to whether it even had a significant benefit.

The story of remdesivir reminds many of Tamiflu, an antiviral medication developed to lessen the severity of the flu. Many governments stockpiled the drug fearing another flu pandemic, but its effect was found to be meek and not worth the expense. And yet, Tamiflu costs less than $200 and can be prescribed and taken on an outpatient basis. Like Tamiflu, remdesivir may be able to have an impact on the disease course, but only if it is administered during a narrow window early in the disease. However, unlike oral Tamiflu, which can be taken at home, the narrow window with questionable results may not be practical for an expensive drug given intravenously, requiring a lengthy (and expensive) hospitalization.

As it stands today, if there is benefit to this medication, it seems to be marginal, and only when given to a specific subset of patients.

While the rise and fall of the NIH-sponsored medication underwent the natural process of human trial based on theory, the media coverage of the "good" treatment, as touted by Dr. Fauci, went on very dissimilarly to the coverage for another medication being discussed by President Trump, the "bad" one.

Zeeshan Aleem wrote a typical description in an article in Vox: "A pair of new coronavirus treatment reports are offering new insights into experimental drugs being tried to treat Covid-19. Remdesivir looks 'hopeful' but hydroxychloroquine has some worrying side effects."

Scientifically speaking, many medications made sense regarding whether they could theoretically halt viral replication of SARS-CoV-2. The remdesivir mode of action made sense, and another medication with antiviral properties, hydroxychloroquine, made sense. However, it comes down to one simple question: not "Does it actually work in patients?" but "Who supports it?"

CHAPTER 5

HYDROXYCHLOROQUINE

Silenced Hope or Dangerous Hoax?

An old, widely used drug is not an obvious candidate to spark and sustain a political firestorm that would sweep up medical professionals worldwide, damage the reputation of two of the world's most prominent journals of medical research, and create questions about the trustworthiness of major institutions. But that is what it has done. Not only has science in general been affected, but this particular medicine has become weaponized in an all-consuming anti-Trump partisan agenda. During the 2020 pandemic, hydroxychloroquine (HCQ) was at the center of a whirlwind debate that started and ended in politicized science and encompassed scandal and retractions.

As most people know by now HCQ is an inexpensive drug that has been around for decades treating lupus and various other conditions. It is a variant of chloroquine, which came into prominence as an antimalarial drug. Chloroquine and hydroxychloroquine have been known for decades to have antiviral effects, as demonstrated *in vitro* against HIV and dengue virus.

One team with the U.S. CDC claimed in a 2005 paper that "chloroquine has strong antiviral effects on SARS-CoV infection of primate cells," though this was also *in vitro*, which is to say, in a test tube.

This CDC team declared, "chloroquine has antiviral effects on SARS coronavirus, both prophylactically and therapeutically," according to medical doctor James Todaro and attorney Gregory Rigano's conveying of the research in a white paper.

So, the concept of these drugs having antiviral properties is not novel. It really isn't even disputed in the literature. In fact, numerous studies spanning decades show how they have the potential to halt certain steps in the replication process of a virus. The only thing unique here is the new coronavirus, SARS-CoV-2, which medical doctors so desperately want to find a readily available treatment for.

Hydroxychloroquine and remdesivir both work to stop viral replication but act at different stages. Not to mention different costs, as the former is 60 cents a dose and the latter—at least with government-subsidized pricing—is over $2,000 for treatment. By different standards, both drugs were being discussed early on—but a fatal error occurred, tainting the course of scientific discovery.

Back in December 2019, doctors on a research team at the People's Hospital of Wuhan University began to notice that none of the patients they were admitting with symptoms of SARS-CoV-2 had the autoimmune disease lupus. A Chinese media site ifeng describes what happened next:

> The research team conducted a clinical analysis of the 178 new coronavirus patients accepted by the hospital from December 2019 and found that none of them were patients with systemic lupus erythematosus. Later, in the consultation of 80 patients with systemic lupus erythematosus treated in the dermatology department of the hospital, it was found that none of them had contracted the new coronavirus pneumonia.
>
> After a joint discussion with the Department of Respiratory and Critical Care Medicine, Department of Dermatology, and

Rheumatology, Wuhan University People's Hospital, it was proposed that none of the patients with systemic lupus erythematosus accepted by the hospital had been infected with new coronary pneumonia. Is it related to their long-term use of hydroxychloroquine?

The results of an ensuing small-scale observational clinical trial, which came out in February, were encouraging, but far from definitive. The use of chloroquine was shown to have some correlation to favorable outcomes of COVID-19, showing clinical symptom improvement of patients with the new coronavirus pneumonia after using the medication. Based on this, experts suggested that in the absence of specific drugs, chloroquine and its sister medication hydroxychloroquine should be considered in the clinical treatment of the new coronavirus pneumonia.

In February 2020, James Todaro wrote, the China National Center for Biotechnology Development had "established effective treatment measures based on human studies."

According to their research, as reported in Clinical Trials Arena,

Data from the drug's [chloroquine] studies showed "certain curative effect" with "fairly good efficacy." . . . Patients treated with chloroquine demonstrated a better drop in fever, improvement of lung CT images, and required a shorter time to recover compared to parallel groups. The percentage of patients with negative viral nucleic acid tests was also higher with the anti-malarial drug. . . . Chloroquine has so far shown no obvious serious adverse reactions in more than 100 participants in the trials.

On February 20, a letter appeared in the international medical journal *BioScience Trends* with the following title: "Breakthrough: Chloroquine phosphate has shown apparent efficacy in treatment of COVID-19 associated pneumonia in clinical studies."

Yet all of these studies took place under conditions where medical workers were "throwing the sink" at patients, trying to save lives. Similar to how the curve was flattened under stay-at-home orders that had confounding factors affecting the outcome (hand hygiene, physical distancing, plastic barriers), the treatment effects of HCQ and chloroquine were mixed with other treatments, introducing bias.

Because of the growing media attention, a reporter asked the WHO in February about chloroquine's possibility as a treatment. *Wired* summarized the WHO's response:

> Janet Diaz, head of clinical care for the World Health Organization Emergencies Program, answered that WHO was prioritizing a couple of other drugs in testing along with remdesivir, and acknowledged that Chinese researchers were working on even more. "For chloroquine, there is no proof that it is an effective treatment at this time," Diaz said. "We recommend that therapeutics be tested under ethically approved clinical trials to show efficacy and safety."

This makes sense. The good news was, if there was some benefit to the use of hydroxychloroquine, the World Health Organization had already put it on its 2019 list of essential medicines, meaning that it was considered by them to be effective and safe for other conditions and readily available.

Saying that a drug is considered effective and safe in one context, of course, does not amount to proof that it works in another context. And every drug does carry some risk.

On March 13, 2020, Todaro (a nonpracticing medical doctor) and attorney Gregory Rigano, published the first widely disseminated paper proposing chloroquine and hydroxychloroquine for the treatment of COVID-19, essentially a white paper touting the effectiveness of HCQ against COVID-19.

Then, on March 16, a team of scientists put out a review of the *in vitro* studies of chloroquine and hydroxychloroquine current at that time, through the *International Journal of Microbial Agents*. It noted that "hydroxychloroquine treatment is significantly associated with viral load reduction/disappearance in COVID-19 patients and its effect is reinforced by azithromycin."

The study was not randomized. It was ethically approved only after it had already begun, and it was not really controlled as the 16 control patients were treated in different clinics, by different caregivers. As such, while it offered some prospects, it was hastily put together and was torn apart by critics for its design flaws. But a flawed study does not mean it is irrelevant, deceptive, or wrong. Such studies often lead to further work: that is their purpose.

An article in *The Wall Street Journal* remarked on the combination of HCQ with the antibiotic azithromycin (AZ):

> These drugs have been in use for many years—HC since 1955 and AZ since 1988. Only the combination is new. . . . The clinical information service Lexicomp lists the interaction between HC and AZ as Category B, which means the majority of patients require no special caution. Long-term HC use can have adverse effects . . . All drugs have side effects, and HC's overall record is safe. Yes, this is an "off label" use. But that isn't unusual, either. One study showed 21% of U.S. prescriptions were for off-label use.

Here, we are reminded that "proof" means something very specific in the context of medical science. Evidence—even promising evidence—is not the same as proof. And *in vitro* is not the same as *in vivo*, just as research conducted on primates doesn't always produce the same results in humans. But promising evidence is also not nil. In between the extremes of incontrovertible proof, on the one hand, and uninformed hopes and fears, on the other, lies the process of research. That process is far from conflict-free or crystal-clear: scientists, like everyone else, have careers and reputations to promote or protect, and huge amounts of prestige and money are on the line. That is one of the reasons why the process has to be secured through peer review and other mechanisms designed to keep science scientific, as it were.

By mid-March, things were about to get very unscientific, though, with respect to research into hydroxychloroquine.

So, how did a commonly used medicine go from being a drug classified as having a "low risk profile" to becoming the most controversial medication in the world and the epicenter of censorship crusades?

At 11:30 a.m. on March 19, 2020, in the James S. Brady Press Briefing Room, the White House Coronavirus Task Force started a press briefing. President Trump began with opening remarks discussing the recently invoked Defense Production Act, as well as updates on various other topics including work on vaccines and therapeutics, where the president made the comments:

> Now, a drug called chloroquine—and some people would add to it "hydroxy." Hydroxychloroquine. So chloroquine or hydroxychloroquine. Now, this is a common malaria drug. It is also a drug used for strong arthritis. If somebody has pretty serious arthritis, also uses this in a somewhat different form. But it is known as a malaria drug, and it's been around for a long time and it's very powerful. But the nice part is, it's been around for a long time, so we know that if it—if things don't go as planned, it's not going to kill anybody.
>
> When you go with a brand-new drug, you don't know that that's going to happen. You have to see and you have to go—long test. But this has been used in different forms—very powerful drug—in different forms. And it's shown very encouraging—very, very encouraging early results. And we're going to be able to make that drug available almost immediately.
>
> So, you have remdesivir and you have chloroquine and . . . hydroxychloroquine. So those are two that are out now, essentially approved for prescribed use.

And I have to say, if chloroquine or hydroxychloroquine works—or any of the other things that they're looking at that are not quite as far out—but if they work, your numbers are going to come down very rapidly. So we'll see what happens. But there's a real chance that they might—they might work.

Most people walking away from this conference felt a sense of optimism that there were treatments showing benefits and could be available immediately, which was more than we had heard on the treatment front since the start of the crisis.

In the very early afternoon the next day, Dr. Anthony Fauci, the director of the National Institute of Allergy and Infectious Diseases, stood in the place in which many Americans had become used to seeing him: right next to Dr. Deborah Birx, a physician who has served as the United States Global AIDS coordinator for Presidents Barack Obama and Donald Trump since 2014. She now stood behind President Trump, along with other members of the newly formed White House Coronavirus Task Force.

By this point in the pandemic, Drs. Fauci and Birx had become such a familiar sight that, in talking about the schedule for the daily briefing, President Trump had remarked that the assembled officials would eventually be "taking some questions with Tony and Deborah, who you've gotten to know very well."

Midway through the briefing, the following exchange occurred between a reporter and Dr. Fauci:

Reporter: *Dr. Fauci, there has been some promise with hydroxychloroquine as potential therapy for people who are infected with coronavirus. Is there any evidence to suggest that, as with malaria, it might be used as a prophylaxis against COVID-19?*

Dr. Fauci: *No. The answer is no. And the evidence that you're talking about, John, is anecdotal evidence. So as the Commis-*

sioner of FDA and the President mentioned yesterday, we're trying to strike a balance between making something with a potential of an effect to the American people available, at the same time that we do it under the auspices of a protocol that would give us information to determine if it's truly safe and truly effective. But the information that you're referring to specifically is anecdotal; it was not done in a controlled clinical trial. So, you really can't make any definitive statement about it.

President Trump then added his two cents:

The President: *I think, without saying too much, I'm probably more of a fan of that than—maybe than anybody. But I'm a big fan, and we'll see what happens. And we all understand what the doctor said is 100 percent correct. It's early.*

When President Trump aired hopefulness in contrast to Dr. Fauci, mayhem ensued. The most twisted and unbelievable medical scandal of the decade began to cascade.

As the exchange proceeded, the president expressed his sense of optimism about the drug, and rejected the notion that he was painting a deceptively bright picture of the situation:

Reporter: *Is it possible—it possible that your impulse to put a positive spin on things may be giving Americans a false sense of—*

The President: *No, I don't think so.*

Reporter:—*hope, and misrepresenting the preparedness right now?*

The President: *No. No, I don't think so. I think that—I think it's gotten—*

Reporter: *The ship is not yet ready to sail. The not-yet-approved drug—*

The President: *Such a lovely question. Look, it may work and it may not work. And I agree with the doctor, what he said: It may work, it may not work.*

The differences in tone and opinion between Dr. Fauci and President Trump are readily apparent. Those differences, however striking, should not obscure the mutual acknowledgment of commonality between what they each said. The president repeatedly expressed his agreement with Dr. Fauci's statement that the drug might or might not be proven to work. The doctor himself reiterated that there wasn't much of a difference between what the two of them were saying with respect to hydroxychloroquine:

Dr. Fauci: *What I'm saying is that it might—it might be effective. I'm not saying that it isn't. It might be effective. But as a scientist, as we're getting it out there, we need to do it in a way as—while we are making it available for people who might want the hope that it might work, you're also collecting data that will ultimately show that it is truly effective and safe under the conditions of COVID-19. So there really isn't difference. It's just a question of how one feels about it.*

Those who wish to bash President Trump as anti-science, and praise Dr. Fauci for being the face of science, or conversely, bash Dr. Fauci and praise President Trump, both need to ask themselves, who is wrong if they are saying the same thing? Is Dr. Fauci lying when he says that "there really isn't difference" between their statements or is President Trump lying when he says "I agree with the doctor"? To be sure, Dr. Fauci and President Trump have disagreements on any number of matters, but this particular question does not seem to have been one of them. Rather, it became an issue because the media wanted it to be.

After attributing the perception of difference between what he was saying about hydroxychloroquine and what the president was saying to a difference in feelings, Dr. Fauci stressed in response to the next question the following points:

> **Dr. Fauci:** *The decades of experience that we have with this drug indicate that the toxicities are rare and they are, in many respects, reversible. What we don't know is when you put it in the context of another disease, whether it is safe. Fundamentally, I think it probably is going to be safe, but I like to prove things first. So, it really is a question of not a lot of difference. It's the hope that it will work versus proving that it will work. So, I don't see big differences here.*

The president immediately followed up Dr. Fauci's statement by saying, "I agree. I agree."

This was not, however, anywhere near the end of the controversy. The war over hydroxychloroquine—several battles of which will be discussed here—continues to generate fresh fury among the combatants. The fury rages on even as some of the key players, including Dr. Fauci, stress the same points: namely, that different kinds of evidence exist in scientific research, and that it is essential to keep an "open mind."

Given the level of animosity toward President Trump here in the United States, it was to be expected that the media would try to cast his hopes for HCQ into the category of snake oil peddled by charlatans. But to the extent that we are able to put aside politics, fairness demands that we not equate legitimate medications with so-called Covid-Organics.

DIFFICULT SCIENCE

It is nearly impossible to know precisely the percentage of people with asymptomatic infections, as they are likely undertested; of those who develop symptoms, the CDC reports 81 percent to have mild to moderate illness, most not ever requiring medical care. So if you study a medication given early in the course of illness or immediately after exposure, the researchers could preemptively "treat" someone with a placebo and it could have the same effect as a medication that truly lessens the severity of COVID-19. Because of this, blinded, randomized, controlled studies would be essential to separate true effects versus the natural course of the infection.

While studies were underway assessing effectiveness for early use of and even prophylaxis of COVID-19 with HCQ, it's not outlandish that when it's already being given in parts of the United States and elsewhere in the world that the president, under the supervision of his doctor, would try it.

In mid-May, President Trump mentioned during a press conference at the White House that he had been taking hydroxychloroquine:

> A lot of good things have come out about the hydroxy. A lot of good things have come out. You'd be surprised at how many people are taking it, especially the front-line workers—before you catch it . . . I happen to be taking it. I happen to be taking it . . . I'm taking it—hydroxychloroquine—right now.

Sean P. Conley, the White House physician, said in a statement later that day that he discussed the drug with the president: "After numerous discussions he and I had for and against the use of hydroxychloroquine, we concluded the potential benefit from treatment outweighed the relative risks."

The president continued, "It seems to have an impact, and maybe it does, maybe it doesn't. But if it doesn't, you're not going to get sick or die. This is a pill that's been used for a long time, for 30, 40 years."

In truth, the president was correct that while the media was in a frenzy over him "promoting" or mentioning the medication, the American Medical Association, the American Pharmacists Association, and the American Society of Health-System Pharmacists released a joint statement in the month preceding acknowledging "that some physicians and others are prophylactically prescribing medications currently identified as potential treatments for COVID-19."

In the same statement, they continued, "We caution hospitals, health systems, and individual practitioners that no medication has been FDA-approved for use in COVID-19 patients." Again, though, desperate times do often call for desperate measures, especially during a public health crisis, and off-label use of medications is not rare, crisis or not.

TRUMP KILLING PEOPLE?

The original message early in the pandemic was that the physicians and frontline workers were being empowered to tackle this unprecedented national health crisis. Daily announcements were made about administrative red tape being cut and protective equipment being provided, but the reality was, anti-science shackles were also being placed.

Following the FDA's issuance of an emergency use authorization for HCQ, the WHO and NIH started running clinical trials to test its effectiveness. At this point, state government officials inserted themselves into the medical exam room.

Strangely, as federal officials encouraged loosening of medical licensing and practicing restrictions, the same caregivers were being restricted by state governments from being able to prescribe medications to their patients. In many instances, state governments threatened physicians with loss of licensure, fines, and even jail time if they prescribed HCQ to treat their COVID-19 patients.

Under the EUA (Emergency Use Authorization), the use of hydroxychloroquine was being restricted to patients who were in the hospital, but that didn't mean a doctor couldn't prescribe it for their patients outside of the hospital. But that is what happened.

If the goal is to decrease the amount of people with severe symptoms requiring hospitalization, then it would have befitted legislators to lift the restrictions and let outpatient doctors decide if the potential benefit of the experimental use of this medication was worth the risk for their patient in an attempt to keep the people out of the overwhelmed hospital.

While there have been reports of inappropriate prescribing resulting in medication shortages in the past, these instances should be looked at individually without universal removal of prescribing freedom, further harming patients from receiving potentially life-saving treatments. During the time of an acute crisis where there are no proven treatments for the offending pathogen, policymakers should have looked to the physicians to make best practice decisions, carefully weighing known risks with theoretical benefit, rather than instituting the draconian constraints that actually took place.

When it comes to the use of HCQ, there are two main attitudes toward it. The first is among the cardiac experts who focus on EKG changes and argue against the use of anything that could potentially alter the cardiac rhythm. I am quite familiar with this group, as a close friend of mine is one of them and I can attest they are quite stringent on all things with potential cardiac influence, including caffeine. The other group includes rheumatology experts who rather focus on the existing clinical evidence and familiarity with the drug, indicating that the medication has been widely used for decades, with millions of people taking it regularly, without mass safety concerns being reported.

However, it was the perceived "what is there to lose" mentality

emitted from the White House that seemingly provoked public outrage regarding the president's comments on HCQ.

High-ranking Fox News anchor Neil Cavuto that day immediately warned viewers on his program of the documented risks associated with taking hydroxychloroquine, saying it could kill people
who are in certain health risk populations. "The fact of the matter
is though, when the president said 'what have you got to lose?' a
number of studies, those certain vulnerable population have one
thing to lose: their lives," Cavuto said.

Not long after that, Cavuto's next guest, an urgent care doctor in
New York City, Janette Nesheiwat, conversely said that she thought
the president's choice to try the drug as a preventive measure was
"very smart."

Over the course of the next couple of months, according to *Newsweek*, "prescriptions of chloroquine and hydroxychloroquine rose in
every U.S. state and Washington, D.C. . . . between February and
March." While 10,350 prescriptions were written in 2019, by April
2020, 108,705 were given, according to the CDC.

Subsequently, according to data provided to *Forbes* from the
American Association of Poison Control Centers, the number
of hydroxychloroquine exposure cases more than doubled from
March 18, 2020 to April 6, 2020, compared to the same period
the year before. Also, data from the FDA reported by *Newsweek*
"revealed deaths of 293 people in the first half of this year [2020]
involved hydroxychloroquine, its brand name Plaquenil, or its sister
medicine chloroquine," nearly four times the number from 2019,
where 75 deaths were reported during the first half of the year.

The FDA then put out an official statement saying, "Hydroxychloroquine and chloroquine have not been shown to be safe and
effective for treating or preventing COVID-19."

The adverse effects of HCQ and its derivates were present
pre-COVID, as, according to *Newsweek* reporting, "in the first half
of 2019, 3,251 adverse events were recorded, with over 2,441 said to
be serious," indicating the person had to be "hospitalized, [became]

disabled or died." As consumption rose in 2020, by the end of the second quarter, "6,588 adverse events were recorded, with 6,233 designated as serious."

Interestingly, though, in the deaths reported associated with HCQ, COVID-19 was stated as the reason for the patient using the medication in "more than half" of cases. The data, however, did not discern whether the patient died from effects of HCQ or from COVID-19. Also, of the calls to poison control, 77 percent of the cases were found to be nontoxic. While it is possible deaths and adverse events associated with HCQ may be overstated, the risks of using these medications exist and they can be fatal. Also, the increased public awareness of these medications was indisputably linked to at least one man's death after he consumed chloroquine-containing aquarium cleaner to self-treat after developing COVID-19.

PARTISANSHIP

House Speaker Nancy Pelosi weighed in on the subject during an interview with Anderson Cooper on CNN: "As far as the president is concerned, he's our president and I would rather he not be taking something that has not been approved by the scientists, especially in his age group and in his, shall we say, weight group, morbidly obese, they say. So, I think it's not a good idea."

Of course, all I could focus on following her comment was that she was incorrect about the president being "morbidly obese." In fact, his height and weight are public knowledge from his annual physical and although he may be borderline obese, he was not morbidly obese. So, I was distracted by her inaccuracy, but that happens quite frequently when politicians attempt to sound "smart" using official medical jargon to garner attention and a false sense of clout. We have had no shortage of that during this crisis.

Kurt Eichenwald, *New York Times* best-selling author, tweeted his opinion on May 18:

> Speaking as someone who has known Trump for decades, I promise you, he is lying about taking hydroxychloroquine. I also expect he will soon trot out some physician to lyingly confirm he is, or will drop the topic and deny he ever said it.

Former Fox News host Bill O'Reilly, meanwhile, echoed the president's sentiment in a tweet the following day:

> If the remedy is useless, so what? Why do [the media] care?

I myself had an endless barrage of friends, colleagues, and random passersby telling me they either support or don't support the use of HCQ, with most of the people having zero medical background or if they did, not having much experience with the medication or treating COVID patients. But everyone had an opinion.

Rather than the rhetoric-filled pundit back-and-forth, there is actually a non-biased way to tackle this heated conversation. Not as a partisan puppet, but rather by evaluating information pragmatically; however, this did not happen.

When you are counting on something as a bailout, it's good to have a healthy dose of skepticism. Unfortunately, while a certain amount of incredulity is necessary, the following events were catastrophic, ultimately eroding public trust of scientific research.

THE EROSION OF TRUST

In Rudyard Kipling's famous poem "If," the speaker of the poem implicitly recommends to his imagined reader that he should "keep your head when all about you / Are losing theirs and blaming it on you."

It is a very difficult task to maintain calm in the face of hysteria or vicious criticism. One of the best ways that we can help ourselves to succeed at that task is to turn to trusted sources that give us access to facts and to wise professional judgment.

It is hard to imagine a desire to make a rather mundane debate about research into a political scandal. A scandal so great that it could lead not one but two of the most trusted journals in the world to publish bogus data as the virus was ravaging the world. It is even harder to imagine that so many highly credentialed people at various levels could have been party to such a betrayal.

In the field of medical research, *The Lancet* and *The New England Journal of Medicine* are two of the most trusted and prestigious journals in the world. Medical professionals, students, and many others turn to them to learn what is happening in the field. Their reputations have been hard won.

In May 2020, an article appeared in the *The Lancet* titled "Hydroxychloroquine or chloroquine with or without a macrolide for treatment of COVID-19: a multinational registry analysis." It was authored by Mandeep R. Mehra, M.D.; Sapan S. Desai, M.D., Ph.D.; Frank Ruschitzka, M.D., F.R.C.P.; and Amit N. Patel, M.D. Doctor Mehra, it should be noted, is a professor at Harvard Medical School and the William Harvey Distinguished Chair in Advanced Cardiovascular Medicine. He directs the Brigham and Women's Hospital (BWH) Heart and Vascular Center, where he specializes in cardiovascular medicine and cardiac transplant.

The *Lancet* study claimed to include data from 671 hospitals from 96,032 patient charts, the largest study to date looking at the effectiveness of HCQ. The findings suggested hydroxychloroquine was not only ineffective as a treatment for COVID-19 but could be dangerous, leading to worse outcomes for people who took it.

The shock waves were felt immediately. Despite it being an observational study and not the randomized controlled trials (RCT) that Dr. Fauci and other public health experts rely upon, the WHO halted global trials for hydroxychloroquine, as the study suggested more people died taking the medication than not.

Dr. Mehra, one of the lead investigators, told *The Washington Post* that it had been unwise to recommend or use hydroxychloroquine and that "I wish we had had this information at the outset, as there has potentially been harm to patients."

"The *Lancet* study rattled scientists testing hydroxychloroquine in clinical trials because it suggested the drug dramatically increased the death rate of COVID-19 patients," Science Mag explained. However, a panel that reviewed preliminary data from the trial weeks earlier did not find any obvious evidence of harm to patients, which is why the study was allowed to continue.

The publication of the study in *The Lancet* pushed Surgisphere, the data collection company the paper referenced, into the spotlight. Immediately after the results were published, the data came under intense analysis by physicians. Many, according to an article in *Science*, "questioned how Surgisphere, a tiny company without much publishing experience in big data analysis, could have collected and analyzed tens of thousands of patient records from hundreds of hospitals—particularly given the complexities of navigating patient confidentiality agreements."

Dr. Mehra said in an official statement that he "personally reviewed the Surgisphere analyses for both *The Lancet* and *NEJM* papers. When discrepancies in the data started to arise, I and the remaining co-authors immediately asked for a reanalysis from Surgisphere and then proactively contacted Medical Technology & Practice Patterns Institute to conduct an independent peer review."

However, Surgisphere refused to disclose the primary data. Doctor Mehra subsequently issued the following statement: "I no longer have confidence in the origination and veracity of the data, nor the findings they have led to."

Let's recap this: scientists trusted a small company to do massive information collection, and while at least one "personally reviewed" the analysis, when that same researcher tried to access it again, the company mysteriously clammed up. These academics, relying on

Surgisphere's suspect data, seem to have unwittingly committed academic fraud on a tremendous scale, sending shock waves through the medical community, at a time when we desperately couldn't afford to make mistakes and the entire world was watching.

Retractions by medical journals, either by the authors or the journals themselves, are few and far between, yet less than a month later, the study was withdrawn from *The NEJM* and *The Lancet*. The paper hadn't explicitly mentioned Trump, but likely the reason for its existence—and perhaps even its underbaked nature—was down to scientists rushing to disprove the president's suggestions. Politics tripping up science, once again.

The Guardian reported that Surgisphere "claim[ed] to run one of the largest and fastest hospital databases in the world," but when *The Guardian Australia* contacted "the health departments of Australia's two most populous states" about Surgisphere's Australian data, the health departments confirmed "the study's results . . . did not reconcile with the state's coronavirus data."

The numbers weren't matching up.

By early June, it had become clear that the harm had been done, not just to the reputation of the researchers but to the reputations of the journals in which the team had published and to the patients who had been deprived of access to a potentially efficacious drug as the result of the use of a shoddy database. The data used had never been vetted, either by the authors of the paper or by the journals that published their conclusions.

Mehra acknowledged that in the haste to publish the results during an ongoing crisis, "I did not do enough to ensure that the data source was appropriate for this use. For that, and for all the disruptions—both directly and indirectly—I am truly sorry."

This is one of those times when an apology, however necessary, really isn't enough. The damage had been done, eroding the trust of the research process.

In a conversation with Dr. Todaro in early July 2020, he told me that "there were too many layers that *The Lancet* study made it through when it was pretty obviously fake." He also suggested the lack of data oversight was intentional on some level in an effort to win the race for academic publication on HCQ.

While the journal wouldn't reveal the peer reviewer comments, it would be surprising if none of them raised any concerns and questions regarding the data prior to publication. This suggests the deeply flawed nature of the academic peer review process—a process that lacks transparency and doesn't allow for collaboration among reviewers that might permit them to build off of or further explore each other's substantive suspicions or concerns.

The *Lancet* paper, however, was not the only source to report concern about the safety risks of the drugs in treating COVID-19. Several smaller, noncontrolled studies also questioned the efficacy and safety of using HCQ. The WHO's trial was designed to help navigate the muddied waters and provide useful information on this ancient medication; however, it was delayed because of *The Lancet* debacle.

The WHO quietly announced it would resume HCQ trials the day before *The Lancet* retracted the paper. But delays had happened and opinions on the medication were now solidified.

The HCQ controversy has shown us that the most highly credentialed doctors at the most esteemed academic institutions in collaboration with revered journals are capable of spreading unverified data. Especially if it conforms with the latest political fad: disagreeing with whatever Donald Trump says.

Large RCT trials—the gold standard to test a drug's efficacy and safety—take a long time for their conclusions to be calculated. However, time was of the essence as it relates to COVID-19. When studies are performed that are not well designed because of time constraints, it can cause rifts.

As we have entered world-record publishing times to compensate for the need of exploration during a public health crisis, we should at the very least acknowledge retractions will occur when things are done speedily. While the world is at war with COVID, publishing data as fast as information becomes available is the right thing to do as people are actively suffering and dying. The majority of retractions will not be from nefarious motivations. However, it is crucial that scientists and researchers remain impartial in their data collection and not allow personal pursuits to jeopardize the integrity of it.

Small, non-randomized, non-controlled cohort studies, and non-reviewed preprints, the ones that help prompt further research, have suggested hydroxychloroquine use *might* reduce the severity of severe illness in COVID-19. Contrarily, the few randomized, controlled studies performed on early intervention and prophylaxis with HCQ have not shown a benefit.

As the collective evidence available thus far does not favor HCQ as being a silver bullet for COVID, every research quest has limitations and nothing in medicine is universal. As such, the anecdotal success reports from frontline clinicians treating patients in the outpatient setting showing success should not be ignored.

It's very, very rare that results are announced at lunchtime and become policy and are put into practice by dinnertime. Scientific discovery is a marathon, not a sprint, with checkpoints along the way. This concept is the essence of the emergency use legislation that was utilized in multiple circumstances throughout the pandemic.

Perhaps one of the most important measures that has been torpedoed during the crisis is the once frowned-upon "Right to Try" pathways, including Compassionate and Emergency Use Authorization by the FDA.

Treatment approval processes rightly take years under normal circumstances to undergo thorough clinical trials and vetting for safety and efficacy, but people with mere weeks or months to live should have the opportunity to try unusual solutions. This had always been a priority for the Trump Administration before COVID-19 existed. When the pandemic began and standard antiviral treatments were having little effect on patients' suffering, the emergency use and other creative measures boosted efficiency in delivering treatments throughout the crisis.

Despite the daily chaos and infighting over issues like mask-wearing and emerging treatments, the government's agreement to subsidize drug companies' clinical trials and manufacturing costs has worked with remarkable efficiency. Nevertheless, despite such efforts, there continued to be roadblocks along the way, altering the already drawn-out process of scientific discovery.

CONTRARIAN BLASPHEMY

Only in the extremely partisan U.S. is data on a potential treatment failing considered good news.

Disagreement between scientists is hardly a scandal, yet the media seems intent upon making it into one. In fact, the silent battle between academia and off-label best practice use is constant in the field of medicine.

Once President Trump stepped into the hydroxychloroquine controversy by announcing he was taking it prophylactically, the political football was up in the air. Everyone started scrambling to intercept it, with questionable characters on both sides of the argument. On the heels of the fabricated data scandal from Surgisphere, a new movement emerged into the forefront, this one composed of physicians claiming efficacy of HCQ and even going as far as saying it is the "cure" for the coronavirus and being lambasted by those with contrarian views.

What we find in Dr. Fauci is not a plan for worldwide domination but rather a scientific purist, with a pronounced commitment to randomized, controlled testing as the gold standard for actionable research findings. He bases his recommendations on the science. His recommendations are formed by his professional judgment as to what sorts of research should be considered relevant in the context of advising therapeutic treatments. As a purist, he needs the data to formulate his opinion.

This is something upon which respectable experts in the field can and do disagree, especially during a public health crisis. For example, while Dr. Fauci will not recommend hydroxychloroquine until there is a RCT demonstrating efficacy (which takes time to do), Dr. Harvey Risch, an epidemiologist at Yale, argued that the use of HCQ in early-stage patients should indeed be recommended, and pointed out that "the FDA has a huge history of drugs going into widespread use in the medical community for decades that have not been established in the basis of randomized controlled trials. Half of the chemotherapy drugs used in cancer were used without randomized controlled trials."

The *Yale Daily News* summarized Dr. Risch's campaign, which started by arguing in favor of HCQ use in the pages of *Newsweek*:

> Risch argued for the use of hydroxychloroquine, in combination with the antibiotic azithromycin, to treat high-risk COVID-19 patients without waiting for further testing on the effectiveness of the treatment. . . . However, of the five studies Risch cites, none of them are randomized and some are on the smaller side for clinical trials. . . . He acknowledges this in the paper, but rationalizes that a benefit as large as the one found in one of the studies cannot be invalidated by the lack of randomization. He also states that the concerns about the sample size are only relevant when statistical significance is not found.

On August 4, in an online statement released on *Medium*, 20 members of the Yale scientific and medical community expressed concern over Risch's advocacy of hydroxychloroquine:

> As his colleagues, we defend the right of Dr. Risch, a respected cancer epidemiologist, to voice his opinions. But he is not an

expert in infectious disease epidemiology and he has not been swayed by the body of scientific evidence from rigorously conducted clinical trials, which refute the plausibility of his belief and arguments.

In response to the profound backlash as Risch did the media circuit discussing his opinion, the Yale School of Medicine put out an official statement that acknowledged the use of HCQ by Yale-affiliated physicians early in the response to COVID-19, but said "it is only used rarely at present due to evidence that it is ineffective and potentially risky."

In truth, our overall understanding of infectious diseases and much of public health has largely not been founded on randomized clinical trials, yet they are our mainstay today.

No one is saying anecdotal and small-scale studies are the gold standard or that it doesn't matter if an RCT doesn't yet exist. It would be extremely illuminating to have an RCT done on patients in the earliest stages of infection, among whom hydroxychloroquine is reported as potentially being effective, but we don't at this time. The question is, under what circumstances can we recommend therapeutics for SARS-CoV-2 when there are plausible signs of efficacy?

Since the beginning of the pandemic, frontline doctors desperate to save patients' lives used hydroxychloroquine across the world. Adam Rogers wrote in *Wired* on March 19, 2020:

Not only is [HCQ] already available, as it has been for almost a century, but Covid-19 patients are already getting it. Montefiore Medical Center in New York has already started seeing the surge of Covid-19 patients that public health experts have been warning about. The hospital is participating in the remdesivir trial and is giving Covid-19 patients chloroquine. "All of our patients get put on chloroquine, as well as on antiretrovirals. We're using Kaletra. Different places are using different antiretrovirals," says Liise-anne Pirofski, chief of infectious diseases at Albert Einstein College of Medicine and Montefiore. "Everybody gets that, unless they have some contraindication."

Many doctors tried to relay their success stories to the public but often were quickly shut down. Other doctors were strongly cautioned against using the drug because of potential changes to heart rhythms as a side effect. My own colleagues across the country have been split as to who gives it to patients and who does not. Those who do say some patients do better on it, and some patients don't. It's hard to say definitively without the controlled-placebo setting, but with hospitals overflowing, time to wait for the trial results was something no one had.

Unfortunately, the polarized environment prohibits logical scientific debate; rather, the media, legislators, and pundits spend more time trying to discredit anyone with the "contrarian" view of a hypothetical benefit to hydroxychloroquine as being "anti-science."

AMERICA'S FRONTLINE DOCTORS

A midsummer video created by the right-wing media outlet Breitbart showed a group of people dressed in white lab coats. The group, calling themselves "America's Frontline Doctors," staged a press conference outside the U.S. Supreme Court in Washington D.C., claiming hydroxychloroquine is "a cure for COVID" and "you don't need a mask" to slow the spread of coronavirus.

It is not ideal for white coats to march on Capitol Hill touting or even publicly encouraging off-label use of a medication based on limited and mostly flawed data. To claim that something is a "cure," indicating it works 100 percent of the time, with no tangible evidence to prove it borders on malfeasance. Further, the physicians in the video fueled conspiracy theories as they alluded that the government was intentionally keeping the "cure" from people to further authoritarian restrictions on society.

Americans should demand the ability to make their own health care decisions, in consultation with their doctors, rather than having media and partisan blowhards who probably couldn't tell the difference between a stethoscope and a microphone influence policymaking.

It is true that public health policy is focused on best health practices to protect people, and public commentary is an important part of molding successful policy. However, while most public health interventions are for the greater good, as partisanship has inflated health policy, there has been an emergency of polarizing intervention, so the emergence of such videos promoting "suppressed truth" will always garner attention and support.

As the buildup to *The Lancet* and *NEJM* retractions were shocking, the suppression of information relating to hydroxychloroquine as a potential treatment for COVID may be another one of the pivotal moments in our history that did more harm than good.

CENSORSHIP

The inciting letter published by Dr. Todaro proposing chloroquine/hydroxychloroquine as an effective treatment was subsequently taken down in late spring by Google after triggering widespread public use of hydroxychloroquine, despite ongoing clinical investigation of the drug's effectiveness in over 100 clinical trials.

The video of America's Frontline Doctor Group on Capitol Hill was also pulled by YouTube, Twitter, and Facebook, citing the following reasons:

Facebook: We've removed this video for sharing false information about cures and treatments for Covid-19.

Twitter: Tweets containing the video violate its COVID-19 misinformation policy.

YouTube: The video met the bar for removal because it claimed a guaranteed cure of Covid-19.

Yet, the removal of the videos by tech tyrants without thoughtful discussion and acknowledgment confuses the public about these drugs. Americans are now aware of the medications, and the censoring of those who support it incites conspiracy ideologies and outrage.

Physicians, patients, and all people alike should be trusted to have a free exchange of ideas with the right to debate them.

Censorship compounds such issues.

There are a lot of reasons not to publicly promote or dispense a medication given well-documented risks. It is for this exact reason many do not support direct-to-consumer pharmaceutical and medical device marketing. Had the topic of treatments for COVID-19 remained generalized during the White House press briefings, people might not have become consumed with the minutia, missing the forest through the trees, so to speak.

An honest and thorough conversation regarding potential risk versus benefit for any medication between a patient and their doctor should never be verboten.

Most people's opinions may not really matter when it comes to whether this medication works or not, yet people are consumed with the subject. As researchers were continuing to study the possible efficacy and physicians were trying to save their patients, the majority were distracted by the political warfare.

By early July, however, the FDA revoked the Emergency Use Authorization of HCQ, citing concerns that the risks may outweigh the benefits.

The NIH, FDA, and CDC have come out against HCQ, saying *right now* the data doesn't support it as an effective treatment.

But that means, given that currently there are over 200 trials look-ing at HCQ, opinions may change. We must keep our minds open as people will be studying this, and other medications against SARS-CoV-2, for months and years to come.

If you believe the government is only out to control us, then you will never accept the conclusions of such agencies once sufficient data does exist. But for me as a physician, I believe in the FDA, NIH, and other health agencies comprised of expert scientists who review studies in detail to give us informed positions.

In my opinion, if studies do show some benefit, it will likely have a small effect, like many other treatments for COVID-19. We have yet to identify the magic-bullet "cure," but even the small benefits can add up to enormous relief from this pandemic. In the appropri-ate clinical setting, sometimes it really is better to "try."

In July 2020, Dr. Fauci said during the course of his testimony at the U.S. House of Representatives that "we all want to keep an open mind" with respect to emerging findings on hydroxychloroquine:

> I will state when I do see a randomized placebo-controlled trial that looks at any aspect of hydroxychloroquine, early study, middle study, late, if that randomized placebo-controlled trial shows efficacy, I will be the first to admit it and promote it but I have not seen yet a randomized placebo-controlled trial that has done that and every randomized placebo-controlled trial that has looked at it has shown no efficacy. I have to go with the data. I don't have any horse in the game one way or the other.

This is about as clear a statement as one could hope for: the data that currently exist do not, by his standards, support an endorse-ment of efficacy in this context. If such data are presented to his at-tention, he will view it with an open mind and, if necessary, change his mind to reflect the new information. It would help if everyone adopted the mindset that is open to change.

Because SARS-CoV-2 is a novel coronavirus, new scientific data continue to emerge every day, whether in research or clinical context. It might seem comforting momentarily to single out "bad guys," but Dr. Fauci or the other members of the White House task force aren't them. Undercutting a top federal scientist only causes further rift. These are scientists, whose focus is on sound data and verified outcomes. Yet, their ability to influence legislators in time of crisis must not hinge solely on evidence-based medicine while negating clinical anecdotes. Without a balanced, transparent discussion, extremes of either *not* trying something with potnetial benefit or trying something potentially harmful will be maximized.

The overall health of the nation depends on these individuals and our legislators.

CHAPTER 6

FLATTENING THE CURVE

The Consequences of Lockdowns

In early March 2020, the gravity of the virus had begun to permeate the United States. On March 9, the Dow dropped to its lowest point since the 2008 financial crisis; on the same day Italy announced a nationwide lockdown.

Less than two weeks later, the United States surpassed China and Italy in total number of COVID-19 cases, becoming the world's largest site of outbreak.

In a pandemic, one of the biggest variables is the behavior of the public. No matter how much power a government has, it cannot control every single person in a country. It's very important, therefore, that the public take precautions voluntarily. People like to feel as though they have control over their own actions in a crisis, and they're often in a better position than a government official to mitigate their individual risk. Big-government one-size-fits-all regulations imposed by force wear on the public's patience and frustrate efforts to persuade citizens to act wisely in a crisis.

One thing we've seen quite clearly is the only thing that reliably causes cases to go up and to go down is what individuals choose to do, and this was obvious from the earliest days of the pandemic, when people saw the pandemic models and decided to voluntarily lock down.

MODELS

Through scare tactics and worst-case scenarios, Americans were being told that epidemiological modeling from the Imperial College of London projected nearly 2 million Americans could die during the COVID-19 crisis if the virus was allowed to go unchecked throughout the population. The earliest model from the Centers for Disease Control and Prevention even suggested the number of U.S. deaths could reach 1.7 million.

The scientific side of modeling is straightforward, but true outcomes vary extensively depending on the characteristics and transmission of a pathogen.

In the spring, attention was chiefly focused on statistical models and what they could tell us about whether the transmission levels would be significant or not. Once that hypothesis was solidly answered, experts then began looking at mechanistic models combining viral transmission features with human behavior characteristics. This is essentially a fancy way of determining "what if" scenarios.

Epidemiological estimates can be useful tools but should not be overinterpreted as we need to allow them to be fluid, accounting for important and unanticipated effects, which make them useful only in the short-term. So, the models of last month, last week, and maybe even yesterday will be wrong, because they can underestimate the resolve of the American people.

The abysmal estimates were based on the reality that Americans frequently depend on doctors and medications to save them, rather than taking charge of reducing their individual risk of illness. We know this because of the alarming rate of preventable, chronic illness throughout the country.

As it turns out, though, it is not only difficult to make a model of a virus with unknown characteristics, but even harder when varying human behavior factors are set in motion, altering the course of viral transmission.

By March 12, a trend report from OpenTable, a popular online reservation system, showed an overall 30 percent reduction of seated diners throughout the United States. In the hardest-hit areas steeper declines were found, such as in New York City, which suffered a 61 percent decrease in seated reservations the same night Broadway theaters closed.

This communal voluntary behavioral change in short order is momentous. While Americans have previously taken decades to modify other behaviors to improve health and safety, such as seatbelt wearing, tobacco cessation, and alcohol reduction, they reacted to the threat of COVID-19 immediately. And without legislative action forcing them to do so.

Utilizing GPS-enabled mobile devices, the private data company Cuebiq evaluated the movement of people throughout the United States, which showed people in every state began staying at home.

The collective data implies that individuals were decreasing mobility *voluntarily*.

However, rather than wait to see the effects of the voluntary actions, a week later, on March 20, New York governor Cuomo ordered "nonessential" businesses to keep 100 percent of their workforce home, acknowledging the decision would cause businesses to shutter and people to lose their jobs. In addition to the business closures, the order encouraged residents across the state to stay within their home as children were also kept out of school.

The executive order known as PAUSE was only supposed to be in effect through April 29 as the state worked to lower the number of cases and allow hospitals to "catch up." The other tristate-area governors followed suit, mandating the entire region's residents to stay home.

While Americans in the hardest-hit Northeast were told to shelter in place, within the next few weeks, many other states issued some level of restrictions despite low viral transmission rates.

EARLY LOCKDOWNS

Think back to the beginning of the pandemic.

Restaurants, bars, movie theaters, doctors' offices, and hotels were closed. Hand sanitizer and disinfectant cleaning detergents were scarce. Coveted rolls of toilet paper were being hoarded or sold on Amazon for absurd amounts of money.

To some, in areas far from the epicenter of New York City, the abrupt actions emanating from state capitols seemed, at least at first, a radical overreaction to the threat. To others who were seeing the recordings on television and social media showing doctors pleading for protective equipment, and families responding in shock to the sudden loss of a parent or relative, it seemed the only thing to do. Everyone who could retreated to their homes. Emergency medical personnel, grocery workers, and delivery services soldiered on. Small business owners put handwritten signs in the window: "Closed for Covid, Take Care!"

Many people relished spending more time at home. No more commuting to work, board games were a regular occurrence, and some even began their novice bread-baking careers. The momentary relief from everyday struggles was welcome for many. Of course, though, we expected this to be temporary, which was why initially spirits were focused on togetherness and unity. But this didn't last long.

By the second week of April, New York state reported more cases than any other country, with over 161,800 confirmed infections.

The majority of schools remained closed to in-person learning as hospitals continued to be full and little information on the severity in children was known. If it was similar to the flu, then children would be vulnerable, so sending them to school could be deadly. Therefore, the early decision to keep children home deliberately bought time—time to compile the base of information that would allow us to make an informed choice about reopening schools, one that we eventually failed.

By the end of March, OpenTable data showed the decline in tristate-area seated-dining reservations to be down 100 percent, and it stayed that way through May.

Meanwhile, the unemployment rate skyrocketed to 14.7 percent, with approximately 70 percent being reported as temporary. How temporary, though, was unknown. And we are all painfully aware that there is more fear from the unknown than from the threat itself.

At that point, we had been hunkering down for weeks, with a (perhaps unspoken) sense that it would be over soon as we were making our way along the "flatten the curve" graph depicted on the cover of this book. At the same time, business owners, food industry personnel, and others sat at home, watching the news, and worrying about how to make payroll and rent payments.

Before the lockdowns were in place, Americans had already changed their behaviors without closing businesses. With harsh orders being enforced, people began losing sight of the collective efforts, as no two people were in the same circumstance. While some were able to safely stay home, making an income and enjoying the increased family time, many others were suffering.

Perhaps it seems that people actually do a better job taking care of themselves than when the government steps in, at least in terms of keeping their families safe. One thing that has emerged quite clearly throughout this entire crisis is that what reliably positively and negatively affects the case count is largely based on what individuals *choose* to do, not what they are told to do.

The country was in a state of shock. As people were home with their kids, government leaders had intervened and were now telling them that their job, their important contribution to solving the crisis, was simply to stay put and for heaven's sake, don't get sick or need any medical care.

Do your part to *flatten the curve*.

Into this state of paralyzing shudder, the federal government launched itself. Though, however you would like to describe the national response to the coronavirus pandemic, please do not describe it as too small. Because it definitely was not that.

PUBLIC DEPENDENCE

The Families First Coronavirus Response Act (FFCRA) was signed by President Trump on March 18, 2020. It was shortly followed by a mammoth legislative whale, the Coronavirus Aid, Relief, and Economic Security (CARES) Act, committing another close to $2 trillion to the relief of the families and businesses hurt by the shutdown. On the heels of CARES came the Paycheck Protection and Healthcare Enhancement Act, which focused on helping small business. These were only the really big pieces of legislation and were only the beginning of the federal bailout.

No one could fairly say that the federal government was sitting on its hands. Everyone on both sides of the political aisle seemed to agree that it was necessary to do *something*, and to do it *fast*. This was fast, and it sure was big. The funds initially committed were $3.7 trillion. To put that in context, the total receipts of the federal government in 2019 were $3.5 trillion. So monies spent in the span of two months during the pandemic were greater than the entire 2019 fiscal year.

Did all of that federal money help? Certainly. Was it, on balance, wise? Did it help the people who needed it most, while targeting the vast amount of outlays to the people and businesses hurt by the shutdowns? Frankly, not very well.

The gusher of federal funds initially prevented the economy from imploding from the shock of the shutdowns, but it was accompanied by a massive amount of waste.

People who lost jobs were helped by checks arriving in the mail. People who didn't lose their jobs also received checks. People who became unemployed received, in addition to their states' required unemployment benefits, an additional $600 per week.

A University of Chicago study estimated that more than three-quarters of unemployed workers were entitled to receive more in benefits than they had been paid to work.

How much more? An average of 45 percent more in unemployment benefits than when they had been working. And this was in addition to the $1,200 per adult and $500 per child that went out to everyone earning less than $99,000 (CARES Act).

Interviewed by NPR in late May 2020, preschool teacher Lainy Morse of Portland, Oregon, was quoted: "It's terrible to say, but we're all doing better now. It's hard to think about going back to work in this pandemic and getting paid less than we are right now when we're safe and at home in quarantine."

At the last minute, a handful of Republican senators, led by Lindsey Graham, pointed out that this provision in the CARES Act was going to pay a lot of people more to stay home than to work, and that this would make it difficult to get the economy moving again. With the upcoming election looming and the economy on the ballot, people grew wary that the Democrats may have wanted a temporary economic failure to bolster election chances and create government dependence. It is important not to politicize blame for responses to the pandemic, but sometimes, people act for political reasons, and we need to be honest about that when it happens—on both sides.

As the pandemic raged on and businesses constrained, roughly 40 million people in the United States had become unemployed since SARS-CoV-2 entered our nation. As though losing financial income isn't devastating enough, it is even more cumbersome for a country where half of the population relies on employer-based health insurance.

During a time when people were needing health care the most, the relief packages guaranteed free care for patients with COVID, but what about those who lost their insurance as a direct result of the lockdowns? Not only did they lose their job from lockdown efforts attempting to protect people from getting COVID, but now they lost their health insurance while still only the people with COVID were being made a priority.

What about everyone else?

An Urban Institute report from mid-September, utilizing 2020 Census Bureau data, calculated that of the roughly 3 million people under the age of 65 who had lost employer-based insurance between May and July, 1.4 million found coverage elsewhere—most through Medicaid—and 1.9 million became newly uninsured.

Rather than helping the newly unemployed with medical costs or job search tools, allotted money went to the hospitals caring for COVID patients and to large universities such as Harvard with massive endowments, yet middle Americans were tossed by the wayside. The average American was being forgotten in this global crisis. While the physical health of avoiding a virus seemed to be the only priority, the prolonged shutdowns caused other aspects of our national state of health to perish.

Before diving into some of the ways in which science has been misused during the pandemic, and the effects of that misuse on schooling, mental health, and the economy, let's remember that initial lockdown efforts were to *flatten the curve*. This was done so hospitals wouldn't be overwhelmed with COVID cases, not to shutter the country in perpetuity.

Nonetheless, by the third week of March 2020, much of the United States had been in lockdown for half a week. The economy ground to a halt. Cases were conspicuously rising in New York City, while the virus spread silently throughout the country as people were fleeing the Northeast to other areas. It was starting to become apparent the initial notion of staying home for two weeks to "slow the spread" was going to have to be adjusted. Certitude was in even shorter supply than was toilet paper.

SHELTER IN PLACE

Rather than groundbreaking 21st-century innovation saving the day, modern-day science played a relatively small role in controlling the virus early on, as 19th-century techniques proved their value. The general truth is that we were battling a 21st-century tormentor with a 19th-century toolbox.

Cities and states hit hard by the coronavirus began flattening the curve by cutting back on the physical interactions that can transmit the virus from person to person. More than 100 years after the 1918–1919 flu pandemic, the same steps that worked against that deadly virus also slowed the new one.

A study, published on the preprint server *medRxiv* in late September, revealed that the stay-at-home measures contributed to an approximately 70 percent reduction in SARS-CoV-2 transmission in New York City from March to June.

It seems like cause and effect when you observationally look at the case counts during and after lockdown measures as though lockdowns directly reduced case counts. However, as FiveThirty-Eight's Maggie Koerth observed, "in the midst of lockdown, a lot of other interventions also came into play—face masks, plexiglass screens at the grocery store, contactless deliveries," and an overall awareness of hygiene to prevent respiratory illness. She continued, "How much of the effectiveness of lockdown was thanks to the lockdown and how much was thanks to those other things?"

As the April 29 deadline for the stay-at-home, business, and school closure orders approached, New York governor Cuomo and others extended them to mid-May. It was also announced school would remain virtual for the remainder of the academic calendar year.

While the pummeling continued, yet another New York–centered pandemic-era crisis began to form: the fallout from halting medical procedures to make room for COVID-19 patients.

CONSEQUENCES OF NEGLECT

After seeing the tragedies occurring in Europe with respect to high fatality rates and overwhelmed hospital systems, it was obvious lives would be saved if we did what we could to make sure Americans had enough hospital beds, ventilators, and PPE to prepare for the influx of critical patients that was soon to come.

Most people *chose* to cancel or reschedule their cancer screenings, routine checkups, and various other appointments as they were terrified by the media portrayal of the hospital and health care systems, avoiding them at all costs. But like the stay-at-home orders, despite voluntary efforts to lessen non-urgent medical care, state legislators, hospital administrators, and even medical societies put forth recommendations and policies to require delaying medical services. As a result, most states in the United States enacted a temporary ban on most elective care from March through May 2020.

ELECTIVE PROCEDURES

Yet, the concept of something being "elective" in health care is quite elusive, outside of the obvious purely cosmetic plastic surgeries. As the emergency departments were overflowing with respiratory illness and general hospital floors were being retrofitted to become makeshift ICUs, state legislators by proxy of hospital administrators flexed their fists and began canceling scheduled medical services.

What our health care system did not do correctly was assume

each case outside of those arriving in the emergency department with symptoms of COVID-19 was an elective procedure, taking away the decision-making abilities of the doctors and patients. Not only were the cosmetic procedures canceled, other interventions were as well.

In early April, a woman arrived via ambulance to the emergency department unresponsive. The woman had been home with her two young sons and husband when she collapsed, and 911 was called.

The phone call first responders received was that someone was dying from what they suspected to be a ruptured aneurysm and needed immediate medical attention. This is not uncommon, as a brain aneurysm ruptures every 18 minutes, with a devastatingly high fatality rate. Most people never even know they have an aneurysm before it happens.

But she did.

The risk of death in a person with a ruptured brain aneurysm is about 70 to 80 percent without prompt intervention, so the goal is to identify the aneurysm *before* it ruptures. In the case of this young woman, her brain aneurysm had been discovered incidentally on imaging she had received for ancillary reasons the month preceding. She was told at that time the risk of rupture of her aneurysm, given the size, was about 40 percent over the next five years. Because of this risk, she scheduled the procedure to treat the brain aneurysm straightaway.

Her initial diagnosis the month before did not constitute an "emergency," in the sense that she wasn't dying in that moment from the unruptured aneurysm. As such, the hospital canceled her scheduled procedure to treat the aneurysm to prevent it from future rupture. Despite pleading from the family and her physicians, the decision to cancel her procedure stood. Two weeks later, her aneurysm ruptured.

While every effort was made to save her, she never made it back home and died in the hospital soon after. Her husband was allowed a brief visit in the ICU, but her children were not allowed at her bedside to say goodbye due to the tight COVID restrictions.

Ultimately, the cancellation of her "elective" procedure, which would have been performed outpatient and not required a hospital bed, resulted in not only an otherwise preventable death in a young mother, but also the use of an ICU bed and ventilator, negating the entire reason her procedure was canceled in the first place.

Government officials and hospital administrators should not be allowed to place red tape between physicians and their patients. We have spent decades scrutinizing medical literature, academic studies, and clinical practice to equip ourselves with enough information to make appropriate decisions for our patients regarding what is best for their care. The last person who needs a say in patient care is someone who has not taken the Hippocratic Oath.

Our involuntary shutdown of medical care was the double-edged sword no one wanted, and we have been seeing the ramifications of such efforts ever since.

People died because they avoided care or their care was obligatorily delayed, and now our health system is being tested as it tries to fix the damage done.

DELAYED CARE

Unfortunately, more selectivity and thought should have gone into the decision of which services were delayed. Certainly, the physicians tasked with the responsibility of caring for patients should have had a stronger voice at the table making the draconian judgments to halt medical care.

A study by the CDC showed nationwide emergency department visits declined 42 percent in April, compared with the same period of time in 2019. While some of this can be accounted for by decreased motor vehicle accidents from people not being on the road, the decline in ER visits underscores a scary reality: people who needed emergency care were not going to the emergency department.

A Harris poll on behalf of the American Heart Association from June 2020 found that approximately one in four people suffering a heart attack or stroke would "rather stay at home than risk getting infected with COVID-19 at the hospital." It goes without saying delayed care in the acute setting will have obvious consequences. For example, an untreated heart attack can have up to a 94 percent fatality risk, while COVID-19 has over a 94 percent survival rate overall. The hysteria surrounding COVID-19 removed perspective into the very real threat of delaying treatment for the two leading causes of death in the United States: cardiovascular (heart) disease and cancer care.

From cancer to COVID-19, early diagnosis and treatment are key to survival and lessening the societal burden of advanced disease. What may be easily treated outpatient requires a hospital bed if care is delayed, which is exactly what occurred during the pandemic.

In May, a Kaiser Family Foundation poll repoprted 48 percent of polled Americans said they or a family member had skipped or postponed medical care because of the pandemic, with 11 percent of them saying the person's condition deteriorated as a result of the delay in care.

CANCER

Estimates show over one-third of Americans have skipped their cancer screenings because the health care facility canceled the appointment or out of fear of contracting SARS-CoV-2.

Research published by JAMA Network Open in August 2020 found a steep decline in the number of new cancer diagnoses. According to BreastCancer.org, "during the pandemic, the weekly average number of people diagnosed with breast, colorectal, esophageal, gastric, lung and pancreatic cancers dropped by 46.4%. Specifically, breast cancer diagnoses dropped by 51.8%—from 2,208 to 1,064."

"Models created by the medical research company *IQVIA* predict delayed diagnoses of an estimated 36,000 breast cancers and 19,000 colorectal cancers due to COVID-19's scrambling of medical care," according to *Physician's Weekly*.

This does not mean that fewer people are developing cancer; it means we aren't finding it yet. When we do, it will probably be more advanced, and more difficult to treat.

Although I did not keep official track of the delayed cancers I myself diagnosed, during the following months my calendar was triple-booked with what seemed to be daily cancer diagnoses that should have been found months earlier. My colleagues and I have begun reviewing the data to see how many cancers were missed from the shutdowns, but the numbers are still growing, and we will likely not have a good idea of what could have been treated earlier until the pandemic is far behind us.

One of my colleagues, Dr. Jeffrey Drebin, a surgical oncologist at Memorial Sloan Kettering Cancer Center, said in an interview with NPR, "Things like mammograms, colonoscopies, PSA [prostate] tests were not being done." At the pandemic's spring heights, Drebin said, he was seeing more patients than usual with advanced illness.

Not only did cancer screening come to a screeching halt, but a study by the American Cancer Society's Cancer Action Network found that of cancer patients "in active treatment, 79% reported delays to their health care (up from 27%), including 17% of patients who reported delays to their cancer therapy like chemotherapy, radiation or hormone therapy."

Early detection and treatment of cancer, and most illness, saves lives. The harsh reality is, Americans tend to lead unhealthier lives than our global counterparts mainly in terms of obesity, heart disease, and diabetes, which is why early cancer detection and chronic illness management should have been a priority during the pandemic. Since many of us are avoiding or delaying routine medical care during this time, hospital systems are caring for patients whose flaring chronic illnesses now require hospitalization and even ICU treatment. As what happened with the young woman with the ruptured aneurysm, the decisions to delay care as people were told to stay home led to hospital beds being used that otherwise wouldn't have been needed.

Uncertainty, of course, is very difficult to tolerate. Small children can't stand it. Even adults have a hard time living with it, particularly for prolonged periods of time. But maturity demands that we not rush to premature conclusions (which might temporarily relieve our sense of uncertainty) that can't be sustained and might even be false.

Ultimately, after many more extensions and last-minute delays, New York's stay-at-home orders were finally lifted on June 27. Like other states in the Northeast, New York flattened the curve. In fact, the goal point on the curve graph was met by mid-May, yet the lockdown orders remained despite New York having the nation's lowest positivity rates.

All efforts to stay inside and physically distance served to slow the spread, not stop it. The goal in America was not to obtain the drastic symmetrical China curve. Unlike China and a few other countries, the United States was not involuntarily quarantining people and locking down neighborhoods at gunpoint.

We were never meant to get to zero cases.

CHAPTER 7

REACHING IMMUNITY

Simple Concept, Complex Quest

The term "herd immunity" has been thrown around throughout the course of the pandemic marking the primary endpoint to this crisis by scientists and pundits alike. But what really is it?

Herd immunity is what happens when a large portion of a community (the herd) becomes protected (immune) from a disease, making the spread of the virus from person to person unlikely. As a result, the entire community becomes relatively protected.

Ultimately, the goal is to reach a level of community immunity so that the country is able to function openly without overwhelming the health systems, leading to otherwise preventable death. But even the simple concept of immunity has resulted in chaotic debate.

There are two possible paths to immunity, both of which we will cover in this chapter: when the community achieves it from natural exposure to the pathogen, and when it does so from vaccinating enough members that the virus is no longer able to spread efficiently (natural versus vaccine-induced immunity).

During an interview on CNN in early December 2020, a newly appointed member of the Biden-Harris Transition COVID-19 Advisory Board said, "Our current estimates are that it would take about

70% of the population being vaccinated. . . . If you have half or more of the population that is skeptical, that is hesitant to be vaccinated, that's going to prevent us from ever getting to herd immunity."

The interviewee implied that in order to reach a level of immunity, and ultimately allow the country to fully reopen, 70 percent of Americans would require being vaccinated to return to some level of normalcy. But that is far from true, as they neglected to account for the growing level of natural immunity.

In the late summer months, Dr. Robert Redfield, director of the CDC, testified to a Senate panel that data "show a majority of our nation, more than 90 percent of the population, remain susceptible." This would indicate 10 percent of the population had been exposed by then and was potentially immune to the virus at the time of testimony.

Yet, by the time of the December interview, the number of confirmed cases from Johns Hopkins Tracking was over 16 million, and by the end of February 2021, it had surpassed 30 million. The CDC estimates for every confirmed case there are up to eight missed infections, so one could roughly assume that as many as 240 million Americans may have already been infected with SARS-CoV-2 by early spring 2021. The 2020–2021 winter months saw over 150,000 new documented infections per day, following the holiday surge. So when people came on the television saying herd immunity may not be reached if massive percentages of the population don't receive the vaccine, they were not taking into account the immunity from natural exposure and that the country was rapidly approaching a time of renaissance from the offending pathogen.

However, it remains an open question whether natural immunity is a viable long-term solution to quell the virus on its own.

NATURAL EXPOSURE

After being exposed to a pathogen, immunity builds in the form of two systems within our body, the innate and adaptive systems, both of which contribute to how our body reacts if and when it is exposed to the same pathogen again. When enough people have this memory immunity, then the pathogen has little influence on the community.

As reported by ABP News Bureau, it was noted during the 2009–2010 flu season that the people who were alive during the 1918 influenza pandemic had less morbidity and mortality from the virus as a result of existing cross-reactive immunity from exposure occurring nearly a century earlier.

There is no constant number in terms of reaching herd immunity, despite what you may see on social media. Rather it depends on characteristics of the pathogen and the behaviors of the hosts (humans). For example, the highly contagious virus that causes measles requires greater than 90 percent of the population to be immunized for an unvaccinated person to be considered safe. Since this virus is quite deadly, vaccination is strongly encouraged. Less is known about SARS-CoV-2, but guesstimates have placed the herd immunity threshold anywhere from 60 to 90 percent.

It's important to emphasize: *We are still finding out how little we know about this virus.*

By summer it was noted that the people who had recovered from COVID-19 and had produced measurable antibodies upon initial evaluation were found to have decreased circulating antibodies several months later, raising the possibility the immunity to COVID-19 from natural exposure might be short-lived.

A study performed at Vanderbilt University Medical Center in Nashville, Tennessee, sampled medical personnel who work directly with COVID-19 patients, and found that 58 percent of those who tested positive for SARS-CoV-2 antibodies in April tested negative only two months later. Even the 42 percent of workers whose antibody levels remained above a detectable threshold demonstrated a significant decline in counts.

The findings were massively disappointing, as they could mean there is only short-term immunity following an infection.

Let's look at the other coronaviruses we are actually familiar with, the ones that cause the common cold. Clearly our human body does not display long-lasting immunity to these viruses, as those pesky colds happen like clockwork throughout the year. As such, vaccine development efforts for coronavirus have been difficult in the past. As evidence grew, half of the medical pundits and epidemiological experts began espousing the need for further physical distancing measures until an effective vaccine is produced that would provide a more robust, and potentially more long-term, immunity.

However, the microcosm of these small studies perhaps does not tell the entire story. Surveillance data from the SARS and MERS outbreaks suggest some form of natural immunity for at least two to three years following initial exposure.

How?

The finding that antibodies fade away after time does not mean the concept of immunity to the virus is lost, despite some eager Twitter comments.

In fact, there is an entirely separate side of the immune system that was undercounted with the antibody and immunity conversation: our bodies produce B- *and* T-cells, which both work to fight off infections and prevent future invasions.

Dr. Scott Atlas, a member of the White House Coronavirus Task Force, appointed months after it was created, publicly contradicted the testimony by Dr. Redfield that the vast majority of the country was still vulnerable by saying:

> I think that Dr. Redfield misstated something. . . . The data on the susceptible, what he was talking about what was his surveillance data that showed roughly 9 percent of the country

has antibodies, but when you look at the CDC data state by state much of that data is old.

The immunity to the infection is not solely determined by the percentage of people who have antibodies. . . . The reality is . . . there is cross-immunity highly likely from other infections and there is also T-cell immunity, and the combination of those makes the antibodies in a small fraction of the people that have immunity.

An understanding of human T-cell response to SARS-CoV-2 and also the possibility of existing coronavirus immunity from our lifelong exposure to other coronaviruses is missing, due to the rapid emergence of the pandemic. The lack of understanding is why most people fit in two separate camps: those who believe we are closer to natural herd immunity and those who believe a vaccine is the only path.

A study published in *Nature* examined three subtypes of patients: patients who have been exposed to COVID-19, individuals who were previously infected with SARS—the similar virus from nearly 20 years ago—and those who have no history of being exposed to either disease. What they found was that samples from all three cohorts had memory T-cells reactive against the surface "spike" protein of SARS-CoV-2. This gave credence to those supporting cross-reacting immunity from prior coronavirus infections. Additional research from China performed on mouse models provided evidence that T-cells are important for lessening SARS-CoV-2 viral load and symptom resolution.

Several more studies from countries across the globe including Germany, Singapore, and the United States have shown the presence of T-cells recognizing SARS-CoV-2 proteins in a significant proportion of unexposed individuals, indicating a level of cross-reacting immunity potentially from prior exposure to seasonal coronaviruses.

Historic knowledge and research indicate that the certain type of T-cell response found present in the research only becomes active enough to recognize the virus when there is a sufficient viral load in the body. Recent mice studies show preexisting T-cells can provide earlier viral clearance and thus less severe symptoms upon infection. Therefore, some experts believe the memory T-cell response likely won't prevent people from getting infected; in the best-case scenario it may reduce the severity of the disease, which may save lives.

So, while T-cells are unlikely to provide full immunity, if they can influence the severity of COVID-19, it may prevent chronic complications of the illness. One can theorize that the high level of asymptomatic and mild cases of COVID-19 may in part be from existing immunity from a lifetime of seasonal colds. If so, while it may not get the country to herd immunity to halt the virus from replicating, it may push us forward to a safer place where the virus is endemic but not resulting in the high rates of hospitalizations and death.

Unfortunately, the data isn't there to confirm this. The data also isn't there to disprove it. Like much else with this virus, it remains to be determined as studies continue to be underway.

Utilizing what we know right now about SARS-CoV-2, which isn't much but is still more than months earlier, we need somewhere between 45 and 90 percent of the population to reach a level of acceptable immunity, while the expert consensus agrees it's closer to 75 percent. Given the severity of disease in the elderly and chronically ill, many more people would die if we allowed natural immunity to run its course. Thus, for moral and ethical reasons, medical professionals have never utilized this approach for a pandemic. Do no harm, remember? At least, do no *direct* harm.

As the discussion of herd immunity became louder throughout the course of the summer, the president's appointee physician Dr. Atlas continued providing a countervailing view on natural immunity, separating from the members of the White House task force.

The Washington Post reported in early September that Dr. Atlas was advising the White House to endorse natural herd immunity in an effort to fight the ongoing public health crisis and lessen the indirect consequences of lockdowns.

During an interview with San Diego County supervisor Jim Desmond, Dr. Atlas said, "There's a pretty good chance that herd immunity requires way less infections because of existing immunity out there. It actually may have already been reached in places like New York. We don't know, but it's possible."

A few days later, Dr. Fauci said during an interview on MSNBC regarding natural herd immunity, "We're not there yet. That's not a fundamental strategy that we're using."

Dr. Thomas Friedman, former CDC director, posted later on Twitter:

> Let's be clear. The U.S. is nowhere close to herd immunity. Pursuing herd immunity without a vaccine would mean as many as 1 million more dead Americans.

While this statement sounded rather bombastic and dismissive, if you were to look at the disaster that occurred in the San Quentin State Prison outbreak and the devastation the winter months brought across the country, you might not find his concerns so outlandish.

As summer came to an end, the California prison system was experiencing massive outbreaks of the virus, with over 16,000 cases within the California Department of Corrections and Rehabilitation. Specifically within San Quentin, there have been over 2,200 cases and 25 deaths among a population of more than 3,260 people. Simply put, two-thirds of the prison's population had been infected by the time the infection rates began to slow. Extrapolating from the numbers, San Quentin's death toll renders a mortality rate of about 767 people dying out of every 100,000. If a similar rate were to occur across the state of California, that would mean over 300,000 deaths statewide. Translating that number to a national level, roughly 2.5 million Americans would die.

Undoubtedly, the unfavorable conditions of prisons do not translate to the rest of the world, as crowded living conditions clearly promote coronavirus transmission more so than the majority of Americans living in single-family homes. However, the San Quentin disaster, in addition to other data, suggests that if we were to attempt a natural state of immunity, it would come with a hefty cost in mortality and morbidity, especially in low-income areas where housing is crowded.

The immunity discourse continued in mid-September during a Senate hearing on the coronavirus pandemic. The following exchange was between Dr. Fauci and Senator Rand Paul:

Fauci: *The guidelines that we have put together from the task force of the four or five things of masks, social distancing, outdoors more than indoors, avoiding crowds and washing hands have lowered transmission.*

Paul: *Or they've developed enough community immunity that they're no longer having the pandemic because they have enough immunity in New York City to actually stop it.*

Fauci: *I challenge that, Senator. Please, sir, I would like to be able to do this because this happens with Senator Rand all the time. You were not listening to what the director of the CDC said, that in New York, it's about 22%. If you believe 22% is herd immunity, I believe you're alone in that.*

Paul: *There's also the preexisting immunity of those who have cross-reactivity, which is about a third of the public in many estimates.*

The interchange between the two physicians was uncomfortable to watch, as they both had merit to their arguments but would not stop to acknowledge the other's. Saying that everyone disagrees with an outsider and dismissing their ideas with a wave of the hand does not improve the state of a conversation. Rather, it further polarizes the issue at hand and closes minds despite truth behind both arguments.

In reality, while the data suggesting cross-reacting immunity exists is encouraging, the data does not confirm T-cell immunity is a prominent contributor in the path forward to long-term immunity. It may be, but we don't know, and we won't for a while. And New York in the winter of 2020 and early 2021 unfortunately proved they had not reached herd immunity, as the state saw thousands of deaths over the subsequent months, with similar numbers to the initial surge in the spring months.

While it can be argued that the goal should be to protect the vulnerable while allowing the remaining population to achieve immunity, the problem is, that would be impractical. The population of Americans over the age of 65 includes approximately 50 million people, and if you factor in those who are obese (70 million) and those with chronic medical conditions (157 million), then generally speaking, at *minimum* 100 million Americans, one-third of the population, are vulnerable to the severe effects of COVID-19.

No one, including rural states where people live miles apart, has managed to keep the spread from hitting high-risk people. So, if the virus was allowed to continue going unchecked and burn through the other 200 million Americans, we may get to herd immunity, but with many more deaths and chronic illness materializing.

Some may still support attempting the natural form of herd immunity, despite that it *may* take another several hundred thousand American lives to achieve it. This potential, however, creates a moral conflict: in short, it would be survival of the fittest and the

San Quentin disaster suggests such a social experiment could come at a heavy, heavy cost in lives.

VACCINATIONS

A better and more scientifically acceptable path to herd immunity is with a vaccine. However, "a vaccine has never been a major tool for control of pandemics," as a paper from *The Lancet* on COVID-19 explained, "because they either occurred before the era of modern vaccines or, as in 2009, the vaccine became available only after the first waves had already occurred." Though, if a vaccine does become available, the trek to herd immunity can be achieved much faster, and more safely.

From the beginning of the current pandemic, there was a public sense of urgency in seeking a vaccine for the novel coronavirus, which grew exponentially throughout 2020. The foundation for coronavirus research had been laid before us for decades, but scientists had lost interest over the years.

Brenda Hogue, a virologist at Arizona State University in Tempe, devoted her career to studying coronaviruses. After SARS, she and her colleagues, like many others across the globe, turned part of their attention toward developing a vaccine. But when the funding dropped off in 2008, she said, the vaccine went into limbo "and we put our efforts into other directions."

Though support for coronavirus research spiked a bit with the MERS outbreak in 2012, the increase was short-lived. Since that outbreak was quickly contained, the disease didn't raise wider concerns and grant opportunities declined further.

My own friend and former associate under Dr. Hogue told me that she left coronavirus research in the late 2000s because of a lack of drug development being pursued.

When research money for a particular disease goes, it's gone, until something terrible happens and people remember that the disease matters. For chronic diseases such as schizophrenia that have neither pandemics nor celebrity advocates, the research dollars never show up in the first place, even if those diseases have devastating health consequences.

In the United States, drug and vaccine development take years of clinical trials, and then the results undergo rigorous vetting from the CDC and FDA, often taking three to ten years for final approval, an accolade only the minority ever achieve.

One of the greatest public health feats in existence is the eradication of smallpox, an achievement that took nearly a century to accomplish.

Similarly, research for a treatment or cure of the debilitating polio virus also took decades, with many failed attempts along the way. With animal trials beginning as early as 1935, it wasn't until 1994 that polio was declared eradicated in the United States.

While polio and smallpox may feel like contagions of the distant past, perhaps the discovery of the influenza vaccine may be more relatable to current circumstances.

It was also around 1930 that research into the flu virus was gaining traction, taking another 15 years until the first successful influenza vaccine was produced. However, only two years later, in 1947, the seasonal variation of the influenza virus was discovered, rendering the existing vaccine ineffective. Because of this discovery, as occurs today, seasonal flu vaccines were designed using data from international influenza surveillance centers to develop a new targeted vaccine each year based on the strains most likely to be circulating in the upcoming season. Essentially, it's a best-guess estimate.

As such, just because you have a vaccine doesn't mean the disease is no longer a threat. With only 62 percent of children and 45 percent of adults in the United States receiving the flu vaccine in 2018, the CDC estimates for the 2018–2019 season, roughly 34,200 died from the flu. And it wasn't just deaths; add to that the 490,600 hospitalizations and 16.5 million people going for outpatient medical visits related to the flu and you get an illness that upends normal life and the health care system.

FLU: A DEADLY "TWINDEMIC"

The influenza vaccine is far from a magic bullet, with an effectiveness ranging anywhere between 30 and 60 percent against whichever strains are circulating during the season. However, the vaccine is still crucial to help lessen the severity of illness in those vulnerable to the flu, mainly the elderly and young children. For example, during the 2018–2019 season, the CDC estimated flu vaccinations prevented an estimated 2.3 million flu-associated doctor visits, 58,000 hospitalizations, and 3,500 influenza-associated deaths. While far too many Americans are still affected by the flu, when the United States has an estimated 728,000 hospital beds, keeping a sizeable amount of admissions from occurring ensures space for other people needing hospital care for non-flu-related illness. The vaccine also prevented an estimated 4.4 million illnesses that year, keeping children in school and people at work.

Two winters later, of course, influenza was competing with another foe, SARS-CoV-2. It isn't that the flu or COVID requires cold temperatures to be present, rather, the cooler weather forces people to congregate indoors where viral transmission occurs more easily. Also, the days are shorter during the winter months, leading to less sunlight and lower levels of vitamin D and melatonin, which can lessen the ability to ward off offending pathogens.

Medical experts began warning of a "twindemic," or synchronized spread of both COVID and flu.

Because the United States' winter follows that of the southern hemisphere, infectious disease experts look to countries like Australia and in South America to predict the forthcoming flu season. In 2020, because the ongoing crisis of COVID-19 reduced physical contact, prompted mask-wearing, and kept children out of school, cases of influenza were drastically lower than in previous years. Predictably, low flu activity in the United States followed, with fewer than 500 cases and only one death by December.

As COVID-19 cases continued throughout the winter, Twitter users made comments about the low flu numbers:

> We are either doing enough social distancing and mask wearing to prevent the flu or we're not doing enough to prevent covid. Pick one.

And:

> Flu magically disappears because it's not part of the BS narrative.

Ignoring the fact that it has been determined SARS-CoV-2 is more contagious than influenza, as it spreads via aerosols and has a longer incubation period of contagious people walking around symptom-free, not to mention the rate of asymptomatic transmission, there is another factor that has resulted in low flu levels. Another convincing reason that may add to why cases of flu are lower for the 2020–2021 season is simple geography.

Influenza viruses spread seasonally each year across the globe because of a phenomenon known as antigenic drift, meaning they change ever-so-slightly each year. Most influenza viruses originate and spread from Asia because of a culmination of perfect conditions for it to do so. For starters, this region is home to more than half of the world's population, so the absolute number of people contributes to a larger amount of virus able to spread globally. Surveillance data show that the virus then spreads easily from continent to continent over a short time span. But this year, something drastic occurred as international travel largely stopped for the better part of 2020. Air

Traveller PH reported, "Asia-Pacific airlines carried only 1.5 million international passengers in October, just 4.9 percent of the 31.3 million that travelled in the same month" the preceding year.

While the flu has long been, and is still considered, a dangerous seasonal menace, considerable evidence about COVID-19 stresses a startling fact: COVID-19 is worse.

So, while a vaccine may not completely neutralize the threat, as with the flu, it certainly helps.

Because of this, President Trump implemented Operation Warp Speed at the inception of the pandemic: a project set to research, manufacture, and deliver a COVID-19 vaccine by early 2021.

OPERATION WARP SPEED: SHOULD WE BE WORRIED?

During the summer of 2020, more than 165 vaccine candidates were in the works, with five to ten entering late-phase human studies by early fall.

Rather than celebrating the success of such endeavors, doubting viewpoints regarding timelines and rushed research emerged. One side viewed the expedited timeline as jeopardizing the safety and integrity of scientific research, while the other applauded the removal of an antiquated redundant process that has been at the center of debate for decades.

When vice presidential candidate Kamala Harris was asked during a CNN interview in September about whether she would take a COVID vaccine once available, she answered, "I will say that I would not trust Donald Trump."

Following this, several governors, including New York's Andrew Cuomo, said they would not distribute a vaccine in the state unless it underwent a review by a group of his own handpicked experts to approve it.

To be clear, the FDA employs and enlists the nation's top specialists to review safety and efficacy data as well as manufacturing information. The people placed on the FDA's internal and external review panels are heavily vetted and highly qualified for their assigned roles. Governor Cuomo says regarding the vaccine, "frankly, I'm not going to trust the federal government's opinion." However, this phrase itself opens a new question entirely: why should anyone trust his? Will there be public commentary on his state's review as there is on the federal one?

Depending on the logic that informs the opposing viewpoints, both may in fact be legitimate. While the administrative burden of bureaucratic red tape in the process of scientific discovery is well documented, not all of it is wasteful. Given that the drug companies' and scientists' reputation will far outweigh that of the Trump presidency, the concept that they would risk producing a subpar vaccine with the entire world watching is outlandish, even for these highly politicized times. To appease the public, the leading eight vaccine manufacturers even put forth a superfluous joint statement that they would not submit for FDA review unless ample safety and efficacy data was obtained. The commentary by candidate hopefuls, governors, and others attempting to undermine the reputable scientific process is distracting and political, nothing further. Laying blame and stirring controversy are hardly productive for people eager to influence policy.

When the country should have been rallying around the innovation of vaccines and celebrating the ability to efficiently produce quality candidates, the political posturing caused further divide across the country, adding to the existing dangerous anti-vaccine movement. Especially since the two leading contenders at the end of 2020 demonstrated a 95 percent efficacy in preventing severe COVID-19, over twice what the flu vaccine offers every year. Still, partisan interference undermined progress, because what good is a vaccine if people are unwilling to take it?

By late fall, a Pew Research poll showed a 21 percent drop in Americans eager to take a vaccine once available, suggesting only 51 percent of the population was willing to be vaccinated. The concern that began emerging by spring 2021 was whether the demand for the vaccine would keep up with the supply.

Doctors, scientists, and other experts have been battling such anti-vaccine movements for decades. The dichotomy produced from legislators, media, and even presidential candidates who claim to *follow the science* while also suggesting a vaccine approved by the FDA would not be trusted was infuriating. More than that, it is perilous, leading us away from the overarching goal of herd immunity, saving lives, and exiting the devastating pandemic. Further, once Americans began getting vaccinated and infection rates were drastically declining, public health experts were initially silent and circumspect on advising people on their path forward. All of this time spent saving lives, yet grandparents were being told they still could not visit with their grandchildren, even after vaccination because uncertainty of transmission remained, despite the consensus it was likely exceedingly low.

The ensuing deficit of consensus among our nation's leaders creates a vacuum, one that rumors, bizarre notions, and a flurry of changing information fill up. The resulting environment makes people confused, even distrustful.

Uncertainty is not the same as panic. Open-mindedness cannot and should not be avoided. Science depends upon it. This is how it is supposed to work. We want our doctors, political leaders, and scientists to respond to new data and dissect it. Normally, we don't witness science while it is underway, in the lab, during the trial-and-error phase. But with COVID, every step is under the microscope of public opinion. In such a setting, you find a rhythm of one step forward, two steps back, or even sometimes two forward and one back. While this is expected among researchers, it is unsettling among the public.

Witnessing the discovery process should actually give us faith in our experts rather than distrust. We don't want these heroes to be infallible and stubborn, but adaptable to learning and hypothesizing. We have to operate within the gaps of our knowledge. This means that sometimes the experts will be wrong.

The COVID pandemic has polarized both sides of the political spectrum with loud voices blinding many from seeing reality, or even acknowledging an alternate hypothesis.

There's an old joke that states, ask ten doctors a question and you'll get eleven answers. A perpetual disagreement between scientists only adds to the confusion undermining our trust in science, but debates over science are nothing new. Scientists routinely tolerate subjects with areas of agreement *and* disagreement. Somehow, non-scientists are unable to tolerate both.

In a time when the country is in the quest to produce a vaccine against SARS-CoV-2, perhaps the real mission should be to immunize the nation against politics infiltrating science.

The pandemic is moving too fast for traditional science and popular perceptions of the same.

Ironically, the devastation of widespread new infections by the end of 2020 provided millions more Americans with natural immunity, so the 51 percent willing to take the vaccine may actually be enough by the time it is widely available. Education campaigns and transparency will be crucial in ensuring enough Americans receive the vaccine, but how many need to be vaccinated remains debatable and with the many variants, a booster vaccine will likely be necessary.

Collective illiteracy and impatience with respect to the history and prospects of medical science are creating dangerous tendencies toward cynicism and conspiratorial thinking. Some scientific researchers, in their rush to publish results, are only making matters worse, as we saw with HCQ and remdesivir.

Given the high stakes, there are going to be charlatans, self-promoters, and well-intentioned makers of mistakes in abundance throughout a crisis. Now is a good time to get informed. It is time to consider different perspectives, improve our collective and individual habits of judgment, and learn to distinguish between productive uncertainty and true grounds for panic.

INFLATED CASE COUNTS

Rushed research may very well yield failed results. But delayed research may come too late. The goal, then, is obviously to find a happy medium. Even when timing doesn't hinder testing programs, other errors can turn testing—a necessary medium—into a vehicle for delivering false results, leaving us blind. We saw this with the lack of testing and not knowing how much of the country had been exposed to the virus.

When it comes to case counts, it is extremely difficult to arrive at accurate numbers because of persistent problems in how test results are being tabulated, as well as problems with the question of how cases are being defined. Some of these problems of accuracy stem from an abundance of caution, while others stem from distortion, either for the sake of blaming some politicians and exonerating others or for financial reasons, as in the case of hospitals that may be incentivized to overreport cases or take on more COVID-19 patients than non-COVID.

As late as May 2020, the CDC was still making destructive errors with respect to tests. As Alexis C. Madrigal and Robinson Meyer reported in an article in *Atlantic Monthly*:

The Centers for Disease Control and Prevention is conflating the results of two different types of coronavirus tests, distorting several important metrics and providing the country with an inaccurate picture of the state of the pandemic. We've learned that the CDC is making, at best, a debilitating mistake: combining test results that diagnose current coronavirus infections with test results that measure whether someone has ever had the virus. The upshot is that the government's

disease-fighting agency is overstating the country's ability to test people who are sick with COVID-19.

Who needs distortions of science by politicians when the agencies led by scientists responsible for disseminating valid tests and data can do so much on their own to imperil public trust?

When we look at the data regarding case counts circulating during the pandemic, several problematic features stand out:

Many presumed positive cases were being tabulated as positive cases when symptomatic people presented who had been to an area with high viral transmission. But the entire country was full of epidemiological spread and it was still flu season, so were cases being overestimated?

In the beginning, before testing was readily accessible, much of this predictive diagnostic criteria was understandable, because it was better to be overly cautious and assume more people had the virus than not. However, by midsummer as cases were increasing across the United States, according to the CDC, presumed positive cases were still being allowed into the official counts despite broader access to testing.

The incompetence continued, as not only were the cases being overinflated, but the number of tests being performed were as well. Antibody tests were being reported in addition to the PCR antigen tests when reporting how many tests were being conducted in a single day. In some states, positive antibody tests were also being reported as new cases.

While a positive antibody test may indicate recent exposure to the virus, it doesn't reflect an active case and may be subject to the quintessential "double-dipping" if it was considered a positive case during the initial infection following an antigen test or even a presumed positive, and then again reported as a case by a later-obtained antibody test.

The problems regarding the tabulation of case counts extend to their interpretation as well.

Misperceptions about facts, especially in the time of crisis, can have dangerous consequences.

For months most Americans would check the daily new case counts, attempting to project what direction we were heading in, while medical pundits were erroneously comparing the United States to various other countries.

On August 4, 2020, Factcheck.org, a site dedicated to disputing POTUS's remarks, wrote:

> The outbreaks in numerous countries have been smaller and led to fewer deaths, even when including more recent upticks. South Korea, for instance, quickly brought its number of cases down after a burst of infections in March and has largely kept it that way, limiting the total number of cases to fewer than 48,000 and deaths to less than 700 by the end of 2020, following their second wave in the winter. Australia's outbreak has also been puny by comparison, with fewer than 29,000 cumulative COVID-19 cases and 908 deaths by the end of 2020.
>
> As the world saw the second wave of the pandemic during the winter months and into 2021, the United States racked up more than 18 million cases and more than 320,000 deaths as it entered 2021, according to the COVID-19 dashboard from Johns Hopkins University. That works out to about 54,500 cases per million U.S. residents, versus 923 per million in South Korea and 1,160 per million in Australia.

While this comparison may seem disparaging, it also can represent a distortion of the facts via problematic comparison and interpretation. How can people compare the United States, with a population of 331 million people and international land borders, to smaller countries like South Korea (population approximately 52 million) and even Australia (population 25 million), an island in the middle of the Indian Ocean? Did you know at the time this book was being written, Australia still had closed borders, rejecting 75 percent of all travel requests, which continued through 2020 into 2021? It is not helpful for embellished comparisons of such without acknowledging the drastic travel restrictions imposed on its citizens and others wishing to enter the country.

The undeniable truth, though, was that COVID-19 was spreading within the United States throughout 2020 and while our response was initially formed as a cohesive, science-based attempt to slow the spread, the subsequent mishaps and politicization that ensued thwarted basic efforts in the months to come.

In addition to imprecise case counts, the fatality rates being reported were using incidence rather than prevalence. Incidence is the number of deaths being reported. Prevalence, on the other hand, calculates the amount of deaths based on the population, meaning the number of people infected in regard to COVID-19. Reporting the incidence of deaths does not give a clear picture of the death rate associated with an illness. This can lead to misjudging the lethality and spurring panic, hence the overestimates of death rates up to 10 percent early on in the pandemic because we did not know the denominator of the equation, how many people had been infected.

The above criticisms of case and death counts are justified. But misinformation has also run rampant. One important piece of information that became widely misused was from a report put forth by the CDC that stated only 6 percent of people who had reportedly died of COVID had COVID-19 listed as their only cause of death on the death certificate. This tidbit of information immediately incited a conspiracy that most deaths being reported were not actually due to COVID-19, indicating the virus was not as deadly as portrayed, restrictions in place were for naught, and the pandemic was not what the government was telling people it was. Immediately, the theory spread on social media platforms, causing "Only 6%" to trend widely. Adding to the momentum, President Trump echoed a tweet that claimed the CDC had updated its numbers to admit only 6 percent of people listed as coronavirus deaths "actually died from Covid," since "the other 94% had 2–3 other serious illnesses."

People began rejecting the pandemic more than ever, claiming the death counts were grossly overestimated. Yet, any physician who has ever filled out a death certificate could have quashed the misinterpretation immediately, if people would have been open to hearing the counternarrative.

You see, causes of death are entered for the death certificate, often with more than one cause or condition listed. For example, comprehensive data on cancer patients show about 60 percent of deaths in people with cancer are from infections (the most common being pneumonia) as their immune systems are lowered during treatment and directly by some cancers. About 80 percent of leukemia patients being treated with a stem cell transplant develop pneumonia, with pneumonia killing 20 percent of all stem cell patients. Another 25 percent or so will die from organ failure, which also may be from direct tumor invasion or less likely, treatment related. Ultimately, the death certificate will reflect all causes of death, so when a person suffering from leukemia dies from pneumonia, their death certificate may list pneumonia as the leading cause of death and leukemia as a secondary cause. Ultimately, though, had the person not had leukemia, they probably would not have developed pneumonia, and if they did, they would be unlikely to die from it as the general mortality rate for pneumonia in the U.S. is only 5 percent. Similarly, someone with metastatic breast cancer with tumor infiltrating the liver may die from subsequent liver failure. As such, the death certificate can list organ failure or liver failure as the immediate cause of death, with breast cancer listed second. Often it is the immediate cause of death that is listed first.

When you extrapolate this information to the CDC chart showing COVID being the only listed cause of death in 6 percent of people, truly, the other 94 percent of cases had other conditions listed *in addition* to COVID-19. These included chronic conditions like diabetes or heart disease as well as immediate conditions that occurred directly as a result of COVID-19, such as pneumonia or lung failure. The inclusion of additional diagnoses, especially pneumonia, on the death certificate negates COVID no more than liver failure erases the significance of a person having liver cancer.

What the numbers do show is the large amount of people dying from COVID-19 with comorbid conditions, something we have seen from the beginning of the pandemic. Also, the people who may have died in their home from a heart attack, stroke, or other cause initiated by the inflammatory response from COVID may not have COVID listed as the cause of death at all, as they do not undergo diagnostics after death unless an autopsy is performed.

SUBSIDIZING HOSPITALS

When New York had approximately 500 confirmed COVID-19 daily deaths, the medical examiner's office reported approximately 200 people being found dead at home each day, a much higher count than the state's usual pre-COVID rate of 20 to 30. This substantial increase prompted the question, were people dying at home from COVID-19 or because they were avoiding medical care for other ailments and dying from lack of proper medical attention? As the year played out, it was determined both were occurring; people were dying who otherwise would not have had the pandemic not occurred.

Underreporting of deaths associated with the COVID-19 pandemic suggests that the true overall death toll may be higher than reported, not solely those deaths directly related to the illness, but deaths that occurred indirectly because of it. However, while the underreporting of cases may be important from a public health perspective, it was the possibility of overcounting that caused more of an uproar. While this is rare, the possibility of overestimating cases and deaths attributed to COVID-19 has come into question as relief legislation provided higher reimbursement rates for any patient admitted to a hospital for "COVID-19 suspected illness."

In the first round of policy changes in relief packages, hospitals were reimbursed higher amounts when caring for COVID-19 patients to offset losses from PPE and isolation precautions.

Stemming from provisions under the Coronavirus Aid, Relief, and Economic Security (CARES) Act, the government was set to pay more to hospitals for COVID-19 cases in two ways:

- Paying an additional 20 percent on top of traditional Medicare rates for COVID-19 patients during the public health emergency

- Reimbursing hospitals for treating uninsured patients with COVID-19 at a higher Medicare rate

Some argue this incentivized the hospitals to falsify data by listing patients as "presumed positive" when testing wasn't available or even in the presence of a negative test, but clinical suspicion remained.

The Washington Post raised concerns that billions went to wealthy hospitals while poor hospitals were struggling to survive, writing in April that "wealthy hospitals sitting on millions or even billions of dollars are in a competitive stampede against near-insolvent hospitals for the same limited pots of financial relief." Banner Health, a nonprofit hospital where the CEO was paid $21.6 million in one year, received $200 million in the relief package. At the same time, many hospitals had been operating during pre-COVID times on razor-thin margins, with many rural hospitals being on the brink of closure. In order to determine which facilities could qualify for this targeted distribution, each hospital was required to submit the number of ICU beds it had and its total COVID-19 admissions as of April 10, 2020.

While elective services were being stopped, it left little to the imagination as to why people began questioning why non-COVID services were halted to allow space for COVID-related patients, as there were plenty of financial incentives to encourage placing COVID patients in the hospital beds.

While most COVID-19 patients don't require hospitalization, PBS reported that "the median cost for any person with symptoms turned out to be $3,045 during the course of the person's infection, based on data pooling and modeling estimates"—a number that is over four times that of the average outpatient flu treatment, as reported by the CDC. Also, the number of days a person with COVID is symptomatic is several days longer than with the flu, with longer hospital and ICU stays when necessary, and more people reporting ongoing chronic symptoms requiring continuing medical care post–COVID infection. All of this adds up. Coupled with the loss of revenue from halting elective procedures and the increased cost of viral testing and PPE required to care for COVID patients, the increased payments to hospitals may not be as unreasonable as some would like to make it out to be. While I can honestly say that I have not heard of or witnessed any direct evidence of malfeasance in terms of overcharging for care during this crisis, I find that there will always be one or two bad apples among the orchard. Do I believe such behavior was rampant during this pandemic? No. But I do believe it made for a great talking point for anyone wanting to villainize health care workers as shutdowns were having damaging impacts across the country and people were desperate to believe the virus was not as serious as being reported.

DRY TINDER

A less promoted theory as to why so many deaths have been attributed to COVID has been that the world was set up for a "dry tinder" year, as the preceding mild flu seasons had left people who otherwise would have died from the flu alive during the pandemic.

It's true, the 2018–2019 flu season in the United States was milder than other years, with 36,400 to 61,200 flu-related deaths, compared to the 2017–2018 flu season, when the death toll was reported to be around 80,000. By January of 2020, there had been only 4,800 flu-related deaths for the season. Since the majority of deaths occur in the elderly, the back-to-back milder flu seasons left more elderly alive, and therefore susceptible to COVID-19. There may be some merit to this argument. But that form of thinking somewhat functions as the defense mechanism of intellectualization. In order to normalize or even allow a level of acceptance for the high death toll accruing by devising a reason "why" other than the virulence of the virus is an attempt to curtail the devastation occurring from the pandemic.

POLITICIZATION STRIKES AGAIN

When we think about the terrible cost in human lives—due to avoidable errors as well as from unavoidable consequences of failed altruistic endeavors—it is easy to become overwhelmed. We have to stop censuring and labeling contrarian opinions as "anti-science" or conspiracy theories when transparent discussions can have positive results. This is when having some clarity and harmony from politicians, expert officials, and members of the media would greatly help. But when we can't distinguish between polarized legislators and non-partisan experts due to excessive politicization, the situation becomes dangerous. We reached that threshold with COVID-19 some time ago.

At a certain point, numbness and a sort of complacency set in for consumers of heavily lobbied news about the pandemic. We knew that public health measures and potential treatments were either praised or denigrated in part depending on the political affiliation of the people making the recommendations. It was often possible to predict the position of a news organization on an issue without even bothering to read or listen to what they had to say. Many people tuned out or descended into the swamps of conspiracy theories. The mainstream news at times offered nothing but political commentary around the clock, interspersed with ill-informed, sporadic attempts to invoke "the science" in support of favored opinions.

Despite the frequent admonitions that our course must be defined by "science," there have been times where coherence was lacking regarding all facets of the pandemic. As we have already discussed, people tried to turn the use of hydroxychloroquine into a scandal due to the lack of RCT studies supporting it, but didn't blink an eyelash about using ventilators and canceling non-emergency medical care, actions that were also unsupported by RCT studies. Science was trotted out when it seemed a convenient weapon to bash opponents and ignored the rest of the time. The implications for the November 2020 presidential elections were never far from view.

To say that fatal errors were made in the handling of the SARS-CoV-2 pandemic as it spread across the United States in 2020 is not to single out a political party for indictment and criticism. There is plenty of blame to go around. The cost is too grave in terms of human suffering and lives to turn facts into weapons for personal gain. To blame a government or the so-called deniers entirely for the pandemic is absurd and implies the virus follows the boundaries laid forth by mankind. While on any given day it can feel as though there is more division than solidarity across the country, the truth is, Americans are united in the fight against this devastating pandemic more than portrayed. As reported in StatNews in late December of 2020, "Polls since March have shown that Americans overwhelmingly aren't in denial: They believe the threat of Covid-19 is real, they are reasonably good at identifying medical misinformation, and they are largely complying with public health recommendations. Compared to their peers in Europe, Americans are more willing to get vaccinated against Covid-19, similarly likely to wear masks, and no more prone to believe common conspiracy theories about the pandemic's origins."

In the particularly egregious case of the lack of transparency regarding New York state's treatment of people who live in long-term care facilities, and the negligence of drawing conclusions from unverifiable data in large academic journals, we can hope that justice will be done. While initial actions by legislators and researchers may have been genuine attempts to follow the science and control the contagion, eventually the lines blurred and the concept of *follow the science* evaporated. There has not been a shortage of blunders in the response to SARS-CoV-2, but public denialism and malfeasance are not major contributors; rather, it is the weaponization of a public health crisis to invoke panic in an election year that resulted in the greatest consequences, which will be felt for years to come.

CHAPTER 8

UNIVERSAL LOCKDOWN

The Fallout from Neglecting Science

So when our Sickness, and our Poverty had greater wants than we could well supply; strict orders did but more enrage our grief, and hinder in accomplishing relief.

—GEORGE WITHER, 1625, DURING THE PLAGUE

Early September in Los Angeles is usually hot. It feels like it is still summer. That is probably because, prior to the autumnal equinox, it is, in fact, technically still summer. Hence, heat is to be expected. There was nothing usual, however, about the temperature of 121 degrees recorded at Woodland Hills on the sixth day of that month in 2020.

Most Los Angeles County schools had gone back into session in mid-August. But the doors of most schools were locked—not just on weekends but 7 days a week, 24 hours a day. The playgrounds were empty. Inside gyms, the nets and balls and other pieces of athletic equipment sat untouched, building up layers of dust.

In any ordinary year, the schools would have been full of kids, teachers, librarians, nurses, cafeteria workers, and custodians—all members of the community. There would have been children ev-erywhere—walking down the halls between classrooms or to the gym or the cafeteria, or going out to the playground to enjoy a brief respite of running around and playing. But 2020, of course, was not an ordinary year, and for many kids, going to school did not mean walking down halls or running around the playground or indeed, any movement at all. For many, it involved sitting in a chair in front of a computer screen, perhaps with an unemployed parent watching television in the background.

By mid-month, workers went into the schools to arrange socially distanced seating in some classrooms. The desks at which two stu-dents would normally have sat were arranged far apart from each other, with one chair only, and a sign on one side of the desk say-ing "sit here." The plan was for very small groups of students for whom remote learning was presenting particular obstacles to return to school starting on Monday, September 14. But the schools were forbidden to open up to other students until at least after the No-vember presidential election.

One might think that the proposed opening date had been cho-sen because it marked some evidence-based threshold for safety. One would be wrong. There was no purposeful medical or public health–based reason to wait until after the election. And waiting until after the election was specifically what was intended.

Dr. Barbara Ferrer, the city's Public Health director, said as much to a group of school administrators and doctors in a conference call, a recording of which made its way to radio station KFI. The "John and Ken Show" played the recording so that members of the public could hear it for themselves. Dr. Ferrer, whose doctorate is in a field called Social Welfare, rather than Public Health or Medicine, an-nounced, "We don't realistically anticipate that we would be moving to either tier 2 or to reopening K-12 schools at least until after the election, in early November."

If the election, rather than public health or medicine, wasn't guiding the decision to wait until early November, what was? One looked in vain for some compelling nonpolitical reason for the singling out of the election as the point after which schools could reopen. Everyone misspeaks from time to time, so if there was some empirical or logical reason why the election should have mattered in the context of the decision to reopen schools that Dr. Ferrer did not mention, it would have been good to know what it was. Moreover, she referred to the election not once but twice—a fact mentioned by Steve Gregory, the KFI News reporter.

Studies are piling up showing the harm being done to children's educations by school closure, so this is not a trivial matter, as we will discuss later on in this chapter.

The Los Angeles County Department of Public Health (DPH), however, was unable to supply a reason as to why schools needed to be closed until after the election. They released a statement that was meant to "clarify" Dr. Ferrer's remarks. It ended up muddying the waters even further. This piece of administrative rubbish stipulates that her comment "was related only to timing any expanded school re-openings to allow for enough time from the implementation of changes to assess impact prior to expansions."

The reaction was fast and furious on social media. One Twitter user with the handle @LeisureSuitLV remarked in a thread to a post from the "John and Ken Show" about Dr. Ferrer's inadvertent exposure of her apparent focus on the election as a factor in public health decisions:

> They are playing politics! All these shutdowns are a way to cripple the economy for political impact. We see what is being done!

We need not agree with @LeisureSuitLV—nor even support a particular party or any party at all—to share the frustration. Episodes such as that involving Dr. Ferrer remind us that we need to think critically about rhetoric and decision-making in the context of the pandemic without resorting to positing sinister conspiracies without evidence.

The conversation turned into a partisan divide where Republicans claimed authoritarian politicians were making up "scientific" rules to influence the presidential election and Democrats were dismissive of anyone questioning their actions, labeling them as anti-science. However, it defies common sense to think that all people on one side of the aisle are indifferent to public health and utterly callous about the loss of human life.

The reality is that the science sometimes backs one partisan position, and another time, the opposite one. But it's become clear that many politicians, for partisan reasons, are resigned to sticking with bad policies instead of admitting when they are wrong. School closures went ahead in the face of science, which said reopening was reasonably safe. This worsened the situation for parents. Overly harsh lockdowns were far less effective and far more destructive than limited, targeted approaches. When the science confirmed all of this, politicians stuck their heads in the sand.

The unfortunate truth is that both sides are going to play politics to at least some degree in certain circumstances. When we spot a situation like that in Los Angeles, in which there is *no apparent defensible reason for the decisions being made*, it is hard not to take Dr. Ferrer at her word that, to her mind, the election is a benchmark and a factor in the process by which she justifies her decisions as director of Public Health. It doesn't seem unfair piling on to point out that scientific data and not the election should be driving decisions on opening schools.

More broadly, we should rightly wonder about the extent to which officials and politicians of all stripes are neglecting science and data. We should also wonder about assertions that either party is the "party of science" with respect to SARS-CoV-2. Let's remember that history shows us two presidents from two parties—namely President Woodrow Wilson and President Dwight Eisenhower—

who did not model active, effective leadership in the context of pandemics.

We have already discussed President Wilson, but it is worth noting as well that Republican president Eisenhower elected not to push for mass vaccination in the midst of the influenza pandemic of 1957. It is tempting but precipitous to rush into full-blown analysis of overall executive performance—whether that of Governor Cuomo, President Trump, or President Biden. At this point in the still ongoing pandemic, though, we can—and should—evaluate particular decisions to the extent that we have enough information to do so.

At least in principle, maybe not always in practice, science doesn't care about short-term, political considerations of reputation, prestige, "being first," or gaming elections—nor should it.

SCHOOL CLOSURES

By September 2020, the country was perhaps a bit less panicked than it had been at the outset of the pandemic, but it was considerably more exhausted.

We knew a lot more than we had before, but not as much as we might have hoped. So much was still shut down, including most schools. But the country was not uniformly shut down. Rather, it largely depended on whether one lived inside or outside a large city, and, of course, the state one lived in. Much of the power to impose restrictions comes from the states, and for the schools, the rest comes from cities and towns.

A survey of school districts conducted in late July 2020 found that just under 40 percent of school districts planned to open schools for full-time in-person instruction in the fall. An additional 12 percent planned to implement a hybrid model combining part-time in-person with distance learning. As the winter brought a massive wave of cases throughout the country, more children went to remote learning as the year came to an end.

The costs of school closures are high, both for children and parents. A Brown University study found that spring 2020 school closures resulted in a significant loss of educational progress, with children estimated to attain only 63 to 68 percent of the gains in reading proficiency made during a normal school year, and 37 to 50 percent of gains in mathematics.

Predictably, the closing of schools sparked sharp increases in truancy. In the Los Angeles School District, many parents of kindergarten-age children did not even bother to enroll them, resulting in a decrease in enrollment of 14 percent. Of those who did enroll, many did not show up to their online sessions.

My youngest was in kindergarten during the initial spring lockdown and as the semester went on, I saw fewer and fewer of his classmates log into the daily Zoom sessions. As adults we struggle with sitting through long committee meetings and lectures; imagine the attention span of a five-year-old. A friend of mine with a child the same age told me that after a while, she gave up fighting with her little one every morning to "attend" school. Through the tears and the screams, she sent an email to the teacher saying he wasn't up for the distance learning and that she can only hope he will be able to catch up on his reading and writing once schools are back in-person, a date which at that time was largely unknown.

Students with learning disabilities or from disadvantaged home environments were particularly hard hit by the closures. Also, many parents depend on the schools to care for their children while they are working and can't afford alternative arrangements. But even with all the resources in the world, getting young children to learn via a prerecorded video session will be challenging.

Educational development aside, the anxiety and social isolation adults were experiencing were amplified in our children as they were separated from their teachers, friends, and daily routines. Children thrive with structure, an essential component of their lives that was stripped away. A survey of more than 6,000 parents and children in the United States, the U.K., and other countries by the charity Save the Children that came out in early May, as most spring semesters were coming to an end, found about 25 percent of children living under COVID-19 lockdowns were showing some level of anxiety and were at risk of depression. The survey found that almost "half (49 percent) of interviewed children in the United States said they were worried, while just over one third (34 percent) reported feeling scared, and one quarter (27 percent) felt anxious."

Were the risks of opening the schools high enough to justify the cost of creating mental illness? Did the science actually support the initial school closings and the continued closure or was it done out of fear? While we can expect drastic measures to be taken early on in a crisis out of an abundance of caution, to necessitate continued action, we need the science to prove its worth.

Initially, we couldn't answer those questions (at least not well enough). We didn't have the data, and amid the spike in cases we had no time to carefully weigh the costs.

When the majority of schools shut down in March, hospitals in the Northeast were overflowing and little information on the severity of COVID-19 in children was known. This deliberately bought time to compile the base of information that would allow us to make an informed choice on reopening schools in the fall.

Later in the spring of 2020, China, South Korea, and many European countries began to cautiously reopen schools as it became overwhelmingly clear children were not affected by this coronavirus the same as the elderly were. By the summer of 2020, data from these countries had given us a broad base of information on the nature of risks. Many European countries, as well as those in Asia and elsewhere, had effectively conducted a massive natural experiment on the safety of reopening in-person learning in schools with a variety of restrictions to limit the potential spread of the virus.

What lessons did this experience provide? On balance, the news was good. Most countries had found it possible to safely open their schools for in-person learning once community transmission of the virus lowered without large risks to children, parents, or teachers.

Exceptions occurred, of course, as outbreaks in Israel and South Korea required temporary shutdowns, but among a broad range of countries, such outbreaks were found to be the exception.

A survey of 15 European countries by the European Center for Disease Prevention and Control (ECDC) provides a summary of the lessons learned by their experience of in-person primary and secondary education. The risks of in-person education can be broken down into 1) the risks of infection for the children should they contract the virus, and 2) the risk of secondary infection for teachers and parents. All schools covered by the ECDC survey implemented limitations on social interactions, social distancing, and enhanced cleaning regimens, with considerable variation across countries.

The health risks to children from SARS-CoV-2 have been found to be small: the risk of contracting the virus was less than that for adults, the transmissibility appears to be lower for younger children, and the health consequences for those who actually contracted the virus were found to be largely minor, although rising for those in their teenage years.

The conclusions of the ECDC survey on the transmission of the disease were based on systems put in place to detect clusters of virus cases within school systems, followed by contact tracing and follow-up to identify any positive cases occurring within a 14-day incubation period. This is what they found:

- Based on contact tracing, secondary transmission of the virus, either between children or from children to adults such as teachers or parents, was found to be rare. Children were found to be inefficient transmitters. Even when infected, they pose limited risks to others.

- Clusters of virus cases in educational settings were limited in number and size, and were agreed to be exceptional events across the countries involved in the study.

Once we had the data that we needed to weigh the risks, the bottom line was that it was clearly possible to open schools in a way that does not expose either students, teachers, or parents to large risks. Reasonable precautions were taken by school systems in the countries surveyed, and reasonable precautions could be taken here in the United States. Vulnerable teachers, children, or parents could need special arrangements. But for the majority, the risks were not large, and the costs of staying virtual were high.

In July, the American Academy of Pediatrics (AAP), American Federation of Teachers (AFT), National Education Association (NEA), and School Superintendents Association (AASA) made the following statement on reopening schools:

> We recognize that children learn best when physically present in the classroom. But children get much more than academics at school. They also learn social and emotional skills at school, get healthy meals and exercise, mental health support and other services that cannot be easily replicated online. Schools also play a critical role in addressing racial and social inequity. Our nation's response to COVID-19 has laid bare inequities and consequences for children that must be addressed. This pandemic is especially hard on families who rely on school lunches, have children with disabilities, or lack access to Internet or health care.
>
> Returning to school is important for the healthy development and well-being of children, but we must pursue reopening in a way that is safe for all students, teachers and staff. Science should drive decision-making on safely reopening schools. Public health agencies must make recommendations based on evidence, not politics. We should leave it to health experts to tell us when the time is best to open up school buildings, and listen to educators and administrators to shape how we do it.

In combination with the AAP statements and the conclusion of international studies, on September 15, the CDC recommended that schools open for in-person learning, and provide supporting materials on effective precautions to protect children and communities. In August 2020, Dr. Fauci also said that schools could safely reopen with precautions.

Yet, by mid-August, the majority of schools had no reopening plans. The schools closed six months earlier; why hadn't preparations for reopening begun the day after they closed?

Time wasted.

Against the best available general scientific advice, school systems across the country chose not to reopen to in-person schooling in the fall. Why would they do this when they knew going to school for children is so much more than just the fundamental basics of education? Rather, it's learning conflict resolution and socialization skills, and building the necessary relationships that will shape our country's future.

Perhaps an influencing factor was that opening schools was seen as key to getting the economy moving again. People couldn't go back to work until the schools opened. But an accelerating economy would help to reelect President Trump and once again, partisan politics may have interfered with science.

State legislators were being pressured by teachers' unions stressing what they claimed to be an unacceptable risk of in-person schooling. Realizing that control over the opening of the schools conveyed a great deal of power, some teachers' unions even expanded their demands for returning in-person to the classroom to include police-free schools, the elimination of standardized testing, and other wish-list items with little or no relationship to the pandemic. By this point few were surprised alternate political agendas were being squeezed into COVID negotiations; after all, Congress had been doing this daily with the COVID relief package negotiations. Shavar Jeffries, national president of Democrats for Education Reform, said it best in an interview with Politico: "No question, there's a risk that some will use this moment to politicize these challenges in a way that simply is counterproductive. I don't think anything that's not related to either the health or educational implications of Covid makes sense."

Further, the CDC proclaimed, "Extended school closure is harmful to children. It can lead to severe learning loss." It notes as well that "disparities in educational outcomes caused by school closures are a particular concern for low-income and minority students and students with disabilities." And yet, unions and public officials, like the L.A. County health director who said schools won't go back until after the election, were stopping children from reentering the classroom. The delay in returning to in-person learning did not cease following the election. Well into 2021, teachers' unions continued with their demands, now in the form of refusing to return to in-person education until teachers were vaccinated. However, the newly appointed CDC director, Dr. Walensky, said "There is increasing data to suggest that schools can safely reopen, and that safe reopening does not suggest teachers need to be vaccinated in order to open safely." This comment was based on growing evidence showing mask-wearing and physical distancing allowed children to safely return to school, especially as suicides and suicide attempts were increasing in our youth. Yet the White House did not support Dr. Walensky in her comments, despite the entire campaign trail saying they would "follow the science"; rather they said she was "speaking in her personal capacity." But is anyone surprised by the White House's parting ways with their own experts to support the teachers' union when, according to the Center for Responsive Politics, President Biden received more than $232,000 in political donations from them for the 2020 elections? This in addition to the nearly $150 million donated from individuals associated with the educational field, according to OpenSecrets.org.

IGNORING THE SCIENCE

We knew what the science was saying, but government wasn't acting on it. Given what we know about COVID-19, coupled with the recognized detrimental consequences of children staying home, the country was desperate to find a safe solution.

Like the many other frontline professions, public safety, grocery stores, delivery services, and medical care could not stop; childhood development, especially in our younger children, shouldn't have stopped either. European school openings and childcare worker data have shown that teachers are not in danger of catching COVID from children when mask-wearing and physical distancing measures are present.

Children are the future and their educators are the frontline workers tasked with caring for their well-being. Rather than being viewed as victims, teachers should view themselves as essential workers tasked with molding the future of our country.

They needn't succumb to the panic; rather, bravely change the narrative.

Some were citing lack of resources to ensure proper distancing and sanitization while others reported a shortage of teachers willing to teach in-person. Teachers organized protests and waved melodramatic signs with slogans like "How can I teach your child if I am dead?" Why did teachers believe they were the only ones risking their wellness to work during the pandemic? Who gave them permission to embrace special victimhood?

There are anecdotal stories of tragedy across the globe of some educators suffering and even dying from COVID-19. Anytime you read a story such as this, there is an overwhelming sense of wanting to protect them. However, the headlines don't tell the full story, as the majority of educators who test positive for COVID-19 are not exposed to the virus while at school or from the children they are caring for, but rather from their own home and social exposures.

That is an inconvenient truth for the narrative that claims cruel anti-science right-wingers want to send teachers to risk their lives to teach in-person. A study of nearly 60,000 childcare workers in all 50 U.S. states performed by Yale University found no difference in the rate of coronavirus transmission between those who continued working and those who stayed home, though these groups took safety precautions (including masking and distancing) seriously and, according to *Yale News*, "were located in communities where the spread of COVID-19 was contained." Also, data from the CDC looking at over 90,000 children in various districts across the country showed only 32 cases of in-school SARS-CoV-2 transmission, zero of which occurred from children infecting the teachers.

Ultimately, the decision to be a frontline worker is not something to be taken lightly. In fact, whether to work during a pandemic is a deeply personal decision. However, the focus should have been on arming the teachers with protective gear and on mitigation efforts within the school, with the ultimate goal of in-person education. Rather, the feeling was that regardless of precautions taken, in-person teaching was not an option.

While education administrators and state legislators attempted to negotiate, the union has a firm grasp in the community. Imagine if President Trump had intervened the way President Ronald Reagan did during the air traffic controller strikes in 1981. After negotiations failed and 13,000 traffic controllers walked out on the job, President Reagan fired more than 11,000 of them who had ignored his order to return to work. The sweeping mass firing slowed commercial air travel, but it did not cripple the system as the strikers had predicted.

In regard to COVID, when it comes to schools, the science has shown few school outbreaks occurring across the world and lower transmissibility among young children, but this was ignored by our decision-makers leading to further inequalities between socioeconomic classes.

Science and fear may have led the decisions for initial school closures, but it was clear the decisions to reopen (or not) were not being led by science.

A Gallup poll performed during the summer months showed that 56 percent of parents of K-12 children said they favored returning to school full-time, in-person for the fall semester. Another 37 percent preferred "part-time school with some distance learning." Only 7 percent favored full-time distance learning. Even among the 46 percent of parents who said they were worried about their child getting COVID, 88 percent wanted some level of in-person school for their children.

How much good was accomplished through school lockdowns? The jury is still out on that question and will remain so until we know more about this virus and the extent to which children serve as asymptomatic carriers. But the evidence we've seen so far suggests schools could have been safely opened.

An easier question to answer is, how much harm has been done through school lockdowns? In short: plenty.

By late summer of 2020, "the science" (if the CDC and Dr. Fauci may be taken as representatives of science) said it is safe to go back to school while taking precautions. Following the science, Republicans were demanding in-person school resume, but Democrats favored the approaches supported by the teachers' unions.

Although the science said there were safe ways to return to school, science was being rejected, with politicians declaring it was for the greater good of public health.

One doesn't need to be a cynic to note that this situation should not have been about two political parties, yet the division was clear—one devoted, in theory, to "science," and the other, in theory, being hostile to it. Yet, which side was the party of science wasn't quite clear.

UNEMPLOYMENT

Another consequence of children being shuttered at home from school closures was that their parents were instantly transformed into homeschool educators, yet without receiving funding or training for their new role. At any other time this would have been impossible for the millions of families across the country with working parents, but even more difficulty was piled on due to the stay-at-home orders: a rise in unemployment.

Every day, countless people understandably go on social media to tell lighthearted stories about or make fun of the difficulties inherent in the task of working from home. Memes, funny stories, and videos about children and pets interrupting meetings—often in a way that seems to make an otherwise useless meeting semi-worthwhile with respect to entertainment value—abound.

People who have the luxury of complaining about working from home while receiving a paycheck are the lucky ones.

The people we hear from much less frequently are the people who have lost their jobs.

Like many Americans everywhere, my younger sister is one such person who lost her position as a result of the lockdowns. For nearly a decade she had worked as an event planner for a large corporation. While the company remained loyal as long as they could, after nearly nine months of continued travel and in-person gathering being restricted, they were forced to lay off thousands of employees, my sister being one of them. Late-night phone calls and text messages from 3,000 miles away offering encouragement and support became a constant in our family following, but the harsh reality was, there was a deep concern for the well-being of her and her young daughter.

My sister, a single mother to a beautiful redheaded little girl, an overwhelmingly charismatic and beautiful person, silently suffers from a devastating chronic illness. While working full-time to care for herself and her daughter, she also battles an autoimmune disease. The chronic effects of her condition have resulted in the destruction of many joints, horrible rashes and scars, and intractable pain, for which she finds solace in injectable medications under tight supervision by her physicians. As such, she is heavily reliant on her employer-based health insurance to help navigate the costly care. My sister would be content going several months without her medication while she searches fervently for a new job, but her daughter has also battled an autoimmune disease since infancy, another one that requires close monitoring. This adds to the panic of uncertainty. While we all feel angst regarding financial security, oftentimes there is more on the line than just a paycheck.

My sister will rally, but for many people who lost their jobs, there won't be another one. To lose a job in one's 60s, for example, or even in one's 50s, unfortunately, is to face the all-too-real prospect of potentially never having a job again.

In ordinary times, some people might rebound by starting small businesses. But what we might call "pande-conomics" has entailed the demise of small businesses—arguably the heart of the American economy and way of life.

PANDE-CONOMICS

By early 2021, the cost of the pandemic had been felt most tragically in lives lost, with over 510,000 COVID-related deaths in the United States. But the secondary costs to many families and individuals—particularly those whose lives were already vulnerable and precarious prior to the pandemic—have also proved to be crushing in scale. These costs include jobs and livelihoods lost, businesses bankrupted, and education or health care delayed or forgone.

Government assistance had been massive in scale but uneven in its effects. Some of those impacted by the economic shutdowns ended up (at least temporarily) better off than they would have been otherwise as government aid has far more than offset any losses. Others, including many small business owners, were and still are struggling to survive. They have lost years—in some cases, lifetimes—of their own hard work as well as their own invested capital.

There was a strong case to be made that those hurt by the virus and by the economic shutdown needed help. However, to put this point mildly, the effort could have been better targeted to help those most impacted by the pandemic. Instead, federal checks were showered on favored institutions and sent out in bulk to the population in general, many of whom had suffered no ill effects whatsoever. Meanwhile, those who were placed at risk by their job or profession—one thinks, for example, of course, of doctors and health workers, but also of bus and truck drivers, and staff at local stores and restaurants—often received little in the way of additional support.

THE HEALTH REPERCUSSIONS OF UNEMPLOYMENT

In line with the developing economic tragedy facing the United States, the country was also beginning to become aware of how long-term unemployment and social isolation can affect one's health, physical and mental.

As our unemployment ticked closer to 15 percent from the stay-at-home orders, we were reminded of a grave reality: based on information from the National Bureau of Economic Research, with every 1 percent increase in unemployment, we can see up to a 3.6 percent increase in overdose deaths and a 1 percent increase in suicides across the country.

Psychological consequences are varied among people reacting to the COVID-19 pandemic, from panic and even mania to pervasive feelings of hopelessness and desperation. All of which are associated with negative outcomes, including overdose and suicide.

As the population becomes increasingly aware of the socio-economic crisis occurring and the lingering presence of lockdowns, maladaptive lifestyle changes to self-treat anxiety and other negative feelings emerged in the form of record alcohol sales, a rise in divorce rates, increased reported domestic violence, and more drug overdose calls. The negative cycle of mental health and negative outcomes directly from these behaviors all can further lead to additional psychiatric conditions.

Importantly, other health conditions may be compromised by abnormally elevated anxiety and internal stressors, including diabetes, cardiovascular disease, and autoimmune diseases.

While the emergence of mental and physical illness continues to be jarring, there has been some improvement. The unemployment rate was down to 8.4 percent in August as many businesses began reopening, many at limited capacities with pricey safety precautions required to open. Yet many more self-employed and gig workers were still out of work. Lines at food pantries stretched around corners and, in some states, for miles. And it had become clear that a lot more than 30 percent of the jobs, especially in states such as California that had already made life for the self-employed close to impossible, were not going to come back at all.

When the federal government was shoveling out money in the trillions, the money went to the people who stayed at home, and not to the people who showed up to help in the crisis. If we wanted to hand out checks, maybe the people who were helping us get through the pandemic should have been first in line? Perhaps the money should have been focused on safety measures to help schools and businesses place the precautions they would need to reopen so that the moment the curve flattened, they would be able to safely open their doors again and keep their businesses afloat. Had this happened, it's possible many Americans would not have lost their jobs, or suffered the severe consequences of social isolation.

However, at the state and local level, the crazy patchwork of restrictions and rules on business reopenings and closures remain.

To some extent, it is unavoidable that the rules vary. For one thing, every area differs in its susceptibility to the virus. Research finds that above a certain level of population density, the risk of contagion from the virus increases. Large and very dense cities like New York City that depend heavily on public transportation are particularly vulnerable. This is hardly surprising. And it was always going to be necessary to adjust restrictions in response to outbreaks of the virus. What may be an acceptable risk with a handful of cases can become an unacceptable risk as the prevalence of the virus rises.

Keeping businesses closed or restricting their operations has high costs, to both the businesses that are shut down and to the workers out of a job. People want to know that the restrictions are carefully weighed, that the costs are known, that the rules are consistent, and that they are based on the best evidence available. They want to know that those rules are neutrally applied, with equivalent situations treated in a similar way.

When businesses initially closed, most people accepted that the state and local authorities who were tasked with making the decisions were at least trying to be objective. But since that time, a growing number of cases have raised questions of favoritism or arbitrary inconsistencies that seem to serve no comprehensible purpose in the design.

State governors have far more comprehensive powers under a public health emergency than most people would ever have suspected. Granted, the coronavirus crisis has posed difficult challenges, so most governors were given plenty of the benefit of the doubt, but a number of incidents have acted to fray public trust.

Across the country, restrictions on the operations of restaurants, salons, and gyms, on institutions such as churches, on outdoor activities and even private gatherings are piecemeal. Part of the variation is that it is much trickier in these areas to say what activities are risky. How risky are they? Does a mask make a difference? Does inside versus outside make a difference? Consistency is key to public trust and when the recommendations change by the day, when openings don't occur despite reaching the goal metrics, confidence in the leadership falters.

THE PROBLEM ISN'T LOCKDOWNS, IT'S HOW THEY'RE IMPLEMENTED

Data has shown that lockdowns do have some positive effects, but the main problems are when politicians create arbitrary rules, flout their own regulations, or impose harsher and harsher restrictions under the science-free principle that harsher must be better. In July 2020, Governor Newsom in California and Governor Cuomo in New York laid down the law about the particular types of food that would be considered a "meal" for purposes of delineating bars versus restaurants being allowed to remain open to serve customers. If the establishment served a "meal" as defined by Governor Cuomo, then it was safe to operate. Micromanagement through haphazard rules does more to fray public trust than practically anything else.

A "meal," as arbitrarily defined by the powers that be, could not include the following: "Food ordinarily served as appetizers or first courses such as cheese sticks, fried calamari, chicken wings, pizza bites (as opposed to pizza), egg rolls, pot stickers, flautas, cups of soup, and any small portion of a dish that may constitute the main course when it is not served in a full portion." Because if you are eating any of those things, you are obviously at greater risk of catching SARS-CoV-2. Only a real meal will protect you. Take Governor Cuomo's word for it.

In Michigan, Governor Whitmer issued a stay-at-home order in April that allowed hardware stores to open, but mandated landscaping contractors to remain closed. Why was it impossible for a landscaper—a job that primarily involves work in the best-ventilated space possible, the outdoors—to safely operate? The governor allowed department stores to open, but with the condition that they could not sell certain items such as carpet, flooring, paint, furniture, garden items, and plants. Areas selling such things must be closed off, said the governor. If you were buying new socks, you were okay, but if you were buying house plants, you could apparently catch SARS-CoV-2. Also, a car wash at an automated car wash facility was not allowed to operate, for some obscure reason.

None of this made sense. Given the inconsistencies in the orders, and the lack of any defensible logic behind them, they were enforced in some places while others ignored them. Americans are willing to make sacrifices. They aren't willing to bend over backwards for the science-free whims of politicians.

Broad emergency powers allowed for the imposition of a set of comprehensive and strict rules by Governor Tom Wolf of Pennsylvania that sharply curtailed economic activity in the state. A lawsuit against Governor Wolf claimed that rules had been imposed in an "arbitrary and capricious manner," inconsistent with available data and precautions recommended by the Centers for Disease Control, aka "science." Certain businesses had been declared essential and allowed to remain open, while similar businesses and even direct competitors had been forced to close. This lawsuit was decided in Federal District Court on September 14, 2020—in favor of the plaintiffs, with the presiding judge saying, "The liberties protected by the Constitution are not fair-weather freedoms—in place when times are good but able to be cast aside in times of trouble."

Even more problematic, there is an increasing sense that those who are most in favor of rigid lockdowns don't necessarily consider people like *themselves* to be bound by such rules. Most famously, the case of Speaker of the House Nancy Pelosi, who had her hair washed and blow-dried in a closed hair salon in San Francisco in late August despite precautions at the time not allowing salons to have customers indoors. Also, Pelosi was not wearing a mask. But those problems did not appear to trouble her. Not to mention Governor Newsom of California infamously attending an indoor dinner party at a swanky restaurant, mask-less, despite the recent orders to halt indoor dining and limit gatherings. However, Newsom was not to be outdone by the mayor of Austin, Texas, who despite encouraging citizens to "stay home and avoid gatherings" during the holiday season hopped on a private jet to Mexico for a warm-weather vacation.

Do as I say, not as I do.

Erica Kious, the owner of the establishment Pelosi entered, watched her walk through the salon via the security camera. "We have been shut down for so long, not just me, but most of the small businesses and I just can't—it's a feeling—a feeling of being deflated, helpless and honestly beaten down," Kious told Fox News. "I have been fighting for six months for a business that took me 12 years to build to reopen," she continued. "I am sharing this because of what everyone in my industry, and my city, what every small business is going through right now."

Most people in this country are willing to sacrifice a lot when it is asked of them, for good reasons, to save lives. But it's not fair for leaders to ask people to sacrifice for rules that, in the end, they are willing to apply to others but not themselves.

The massive power of the states to impose rules in the interests of public health has rarely before been so severely tested.

Arguably, many rules were put in place without valid foundation in scientific evidence, or a clear link to a public health rationale. It is wrong to demand that people accept a meaningless sacrifice.

It is true that lockdowns have some benefits, but the key is moderation. David R. Henderson and Jonathan Lipow broke it down in an article in *The Wall Street Journal* in June 2020:

> A team of economists from the University of California, Berkeley carefully evaluated empirical data on social distancing, shelter-in-place orders, and lives saved. To measure the impact of social distancing, they gathered data from cellphones on travel patterns, foot traffic in nonessential businesses, and personal interactions.
>
> Their findings? Social-distancing measures reduced person-to-person contact by about 50%, likely saving over 60,000

lives, while harsher shelter-in-place and business closure rules reduced contact by only an additional 5%.

Rather than validating draconian lockdown orders, the latest economic research on COVID-19 suggests shelter-in-place measures in particular, may have done more harm than good. That doesn't mean, of course, that all such measures should be abandoned.

"To socially distance or not to socially distance" is actually not the question. The question should be, what policies actually make sense?

They went on to summarize an MIT study that "concluded that twice as many lives could be saved if governments focused limited resources on protecting the most vulnerable people rather than squandering them on those who seem to face almost no risk, such as children." Of note, the authors of the Berkeley research also concluded that they "did not find strong evidence that some other policies, such as school closings, significantly flattened the curve."

We have to do the best we can with the limited information that we have in the moment.

In the beginning of the pandemic, before testing was available and much was known about the illness, short-term stay-at-home orders were key to slowing the spread. But out of fear, not science, they were prolonged and the country was forced into a state of social isolation and resultant transient economic despair.

The question is, when new information emerges, how can we guarantee our legislators will swallow their pride, acknowledge the measures were in haste, and swiftly rectify them? Unfortunately, they repeated their actions as the dramatic second wave occurred during the winter months and into the New Year.

REFUSING TO BACK DOWN FROM BAD RULES

The position of Democratic governors and much of the media quickly coalesced around a conclusion that the more restrictions, the better. This was understandable in March of 2020 when the caseloads in New York City were skyrocketing daily and hospitals and morgues were stressed to the breaking point. With the threat of exponential spread, there was no time and there was not enough information. Facing possible catastrophe, political leaders had no choice but to use the bluntest possible instruments to gain control over the spread of the virus.

And so, the fateful choice was made: shut down travel, schools, churches, public gatherings of every sort, and close businesses. Hospitals and medical providers shut down all elective treatment to prepare for an onslaught of patients. And while the estimated needs for ventilators and hospital beds did not live up to reality, the evidence began to grow that the shutdowns carried heavy costs in lost jobs, mental health, and missed education.

With hindsight and a comparison of the experience of areas with varying restrictions, it is now clear the shutdowns outside of the New York City area were probably harsher than necessary. They should have known better. The country saw what was happening in the Northeast and, out of an abundance of caution, followed suit. But in the intervening months, the stoppage became ever more tightly intertwined with political considerations. The possibility of objectively using information on tradeoffs between costs and benefits became ever more difficult. Always hovering in the background was the knowledge that the economic consequences of the shutdowns would hurt the prospects of the Republicans and help those of the Democrats, and that the issue of the management of the pandemic would weigh heavily. The coverage of both health and economic consequences became more and more clearly politicized.

Political parties are not competent to pronounce upon the question of whether a given scientific issue is "settled." It would be nice for politicians and officials if all scientific questions were settled, so that unambiguous findings could then be translated into policy and action without delay, but that is not how science works. It doesn't exist to generate claims that politicians and officials can use to back up their policy preferences. Science can't be hostage to the political lust for easy answers and quick fixes, with heroes on the one side and antiheroes on the other. And, by the same token, political devices, such as election cycles, shouldn't be used to influence decisions regarding public health that should depend upon science.

Under the constraints of the pandemic, both parties explicitly depend upon and deploy science. The questions are: how well and with respect to which issues?

With respect to particular decisions, the question should not be "To what party does the decision-maker belong?" but rather "What is the underlying justification for the decision?" and "Does data exist that suggests that decisions should be reversed or amended?"

Unfortunately, this has not been the approach of public health officials, as was demonstrated when the Los Angeles Public Health Department announced all dining, indoors and outdoors, would halt. When reporters challenged the decision to close, explaining that businesses would not survive and demanding to know the safety data that was driving the decision, a Public Health officer cited a CDC study linking dining to a rise in cases. However, here is the thing about that study: even though it was a surveillance study, all it concluded was that people who tested positive with COVID-19 were twice as likely to have dined out recently. It did not say the infection was contracted while dining; it didn't even specify whether people were indoors or outdoors. All it did was demonstrate a correlation, certainly not a causation between dining and viral risk. In fact, strong scientific data show outdoor dining has *not* contributed to a rise in cases. More specifically in the case of L.A. County, restaurants have been linked to less than 4 percent of all outbreaks.

A national shutdown is not a sustainable solution. Neither are localized measures that hurt people, not backed by science. That means, absent a vaccine or effective COVID-19 treatment, reopenings should have occurred with safety measures in place.

Schools shouldn't have closed. Teachers' unions shouldn't have been allowed to bully politicians into enforcing anti-science policies. School closures immeasurably worsened the lot of overburdened working and unemployed parents who suddenly had to figure out how to effectively homeschool their children during a pandemic. And overly harsh lockdowns made things worse.

We needed measured, moderate lockdowns. Crowd restrictions, social distancing actions, and healthy behaviors don't just lower disease mortality, they actually can reduce a pandemic's long-term adverse economic effects. However, they only do this when the measures are limited, constantly scrutinized, and certainly not drawn out.

Reopening measures should be aggressively pursued once a locality has successfully slowed the rate of new infections, hospital capacity is manageable, and effective outpatient testing is in place. This was achieved early in the crisis, yet lockdowns remained. As the second wave approached, the country was restless and suffering. Still the lockdowns remained.

Unlike the secular stagnation that plagued America during the Great Depression, our country was champing at the bit to reopen, with people even protesting to be able to leave their homes again and business owners defying closure orders.

As the economic uncertainty and ruin began its mending in 2021, the lingering effects of lapsed education, prolonged loneliness, and social unrest, let alone the fear and risk of illness and death, will continue to be seen.

CHAPTER 9

THE ORIGIN OF SARS-COV-2

We often hear the term "scientific consensus" being used when people are trying to establish an authoritative basis for forming public policy. Follow the "scientific consensus." Respect "the science." This is a bit ironic since there is rarely consensus among actual researchers, especially with a brand-new discovery.

One area where the science was and remains contested is the question of the origin of SARS-CoV-2. Where did it come from? Early rumors distributed by Chinese authorities have remained largely unchallenged. This is a mistake.

Dr. Zhong Nanshan is a well-known Chinese physician, made famous for his work and public messaging during the first SARS outbreak. In 2020, the 84-year-old medical doctor and fitness guru returned to the spotlight when he asserted that "though the virus was first discovered in China, it may *not* have originated there." The statement, seemingly simple and innocent aside, had profound consequences as his words were used by the Chinese government to fuel a litany of conspiracy theories.

Shortly after his pronouncement, Chinese officials eagerly latched onto the idea and began floating the rumor the novel coronavirus may have been brought to China from elsewhere, more specifically, the United States. On March 12, 2020, Chinese Foreign

Ministry spokesman Zhao Lijian wrote (in English) on his Twitter account:

> When did patient zero begin in US? How many people are infected? What are the names of the hospitals? It might be US army who brought the epidemic to Wuhan. Be transparent! Make public your data! US owe us an explanation!

The Chinese Ministry spokesperson was referring to debunked conjecture by media personality George Webb, who in a series of YouTube videos branded Maatje Benassi, a female army reservist who traveled to Wuhan in October 2019 to compete as a cyclist in the 2019 Military World Games, as Patient Zero. Benassi "collapsed" during the 50-mile cycling race and, Webb claimed, showed some other "typical symptoms of coronavirus." He then made the leap that since Maatje's husband worked near an area in Virginia that had a "mystery illness" outbreak during the summer of 2019, he was the connection. He surmised that Benassi's husband contracted the virus and gave it to his wife, who then brought it to Wuhan several months later during the competition.

There are several problems with this theory. For one thing, the "mystery illness" is no longer a mystery. True, during June and July of 2019 there were localized flu-like outbreaks in a few surrounding nursing homes in Northern Virginia, sending many to the hospital and even resulting in three deaths.

But the Fairfax Health Department performed an investigation of the outbreak, with their final update posted on July 29, 2019:

> No new cases of illness have occurred in Heatherwood since July 15, 2019. Results of earlier testing submitted to the Centers for Disease Control and Prevention indicated *rhinovirus*, a virus that causes the common cold. The facility continues normal operations.

As exotic as it may sound, rhinovirus, like a coronavirus, is a common cause of upper and lower respiratory tract infections in adults, and is associated with significantly higher mortality in institutionalized older adults, such as nursing home residents. Unlike the coronavirus, rhinovirus has more fomite (hand-to-mouth) transmission than aerosol, making it easier to contain. Again, had this "mystery illness" been the novel coronavirus, which is proving to be the most contagious and difficult-to-contain coronavirus in history, it is *highly* unlikely it would have halted in Northern Virginia, only to travel to Wuhan without spreading elsewhere first.

As if that wasn't enough to put an end to his notion, the true account by Maatje, fellow cyclists, and onlookers at the military athletic event describe the incident in question as a collision among cyclists. As Maatje made a turn, her competitor's front tire hit her back tire, causing the bike to buckle beneath her. When Maatje "collapsed" to the ground, the collision literally knocked the wind out of her. "I just had to catch my breath, but it wouldn't come," Maatje said to journalists following the race. However, she was able to get back on her bike to finish the race, later being diagnosed with a concussion and broken ribs, explaining her symptoms of being short of breath.

Despite this, posts inferring the U.S. military athlete may have brought the virus to Wuhan have still not been removed by China's strict internet censors. This suggests that these conspiracies fit closely with the obscurantist goals of the Chinese government, as they are usually quick to remove information they deem to be "misinformation."

Such efforts to deceive exist despite the vast amount of information that leads us to suspect a Chinese origin for the virus. Even Dr. Zhong Nanshan wrote a paper over a decade earlier following the 2003 SARS outbreak, where he described lessons learned from the experience and warned: "Wildlife markets represent a dangerous source of possible new infections that could undermine the prevention of SARS . . . If no action is taken to control wildlife markets, the SARS-CoV organism may develop into an epidemic strain."

He also explained that the Chinese government covered up that outbreak, writing, "The first case of SARS appeared in Guangdong province, China, in November 2002, but information about it was not broadcast on Central TV, the official Chinese television station, until February 2003, though rumors spread via cell phones and the internet. It was not until three months after the breakout of epidemics that a group of healthcare officials were sent to investigate. Before this, the absence of open news was an attempt to maintain social stability."

Finally, he detailed the cases of several lab employees who spread SARS outside the lab. Such mistakes occurred in labs that disregarded regulations, "allowing non-professionals to be on SARS research projects; downplaying biosafety regulations; using methods with unconfirmed efficacy to inactivate viruses . . . delay in monitoring fever, etc."

He practically outlined all of the likely reasons there would be an outbreak in China, from wet markets to negligence at labs.

Another prediction of a future outbreak originating in China appeared in the abstract of a paper published by scientists at the Wuhan Institute of Virology in March 2019, where they noted "it is highly likely that future SARS- or MERS-like coronavirus outbreaks will originate from bats, and there is an increased probability that this will occur in China."

This simple acknowledgment—which came directly from the Wuhan Institute of Virology—coupled with Dr. Zhong's foresight on wildlife "wet" markets, lab safety concerns, and concealment efforts by the Chinese Communist Party (CCP) makes one wonder how, according to a May 2020 article in *The Wall Street Journal*, China has continued to deny both the Wuhan market and the Wuhan Institute of Virology as points of origin for the novel coronavirus. The answer, of course, is that China isn't actually trying to rule them out because it doesn't want to be responsible for the deadly pandemic.

Absent a miraculous change of heart from this authoritarian regime, there is no sign that a common understanding can be reached between China and the rest of the world regarding the origins of the virus. Yet such an understanding is necessary to save lives globally as the politicization of the virus becomes deadly.

The fight against the virus is often just as much a fight for accurate information and wise public health guidance. Lacking an apparent scientific consensus or reliable data (which are not the same thing in science) about the nature of the virus, we end up with warring personal opinions. This is dangerous territory when it comes to pandemics. It can result in the impression that science is another arena in which people cannot get their stories straight and in which the perceived discord results in public panic and ultimately, suppression of opinions that appear to be contrarian.

In a democratic system of governance such as ours, we are influenced by consensus in the form of majority rule. When it comes to science, we crave consensus in evidence-based medicine, because it confers legitimacy and provides a way to shut down minority opinions, which include superstitions and outlandish speculations. But science that challenges the consensus in responsible ways, while it may be unpopular, can be vital to advancement.

So how do we distinguish false rumors from unpopular opinions that might have some measure of the truth?

We follow the evidence. Start at the beginning. How did this pandemic commence? A basic question that still has not been answered.

CORONAVIRIDAE: A HISTORY OF DEADLY CORONAVIRUSES

Coronaviridae is a big family of different types of coronavirus.

The name "corona" comes from the crown-like appearance of S "spike" proteins on the surface of the virus itself. The most common human coronavirus (CoV) causes the "common cold," first identified in 1965 when Tyrrell and Bynoe cultured a virus from the respiratory tract of an adult. Other, less commonly known types mostly infect animals, including bats, camels, and cattle.

As our knowledge of virology and pathogenicity has grown over the last century, nothing has been more predictable than the emergence of new diseases. Since 2003, at least five new human coronaviruses have been identified. In the last two decades alone, prior to 2020, we have had two major outbreaks from them: Severe Acute Respiratory Syndrome (SARS) and Middle East Respiratory Syndrome (MERS).

Beginning in 2002, SARS swept through China before it was identified in early 2003 and proceeded to spread to 28 other countries. More than 8,000 people were infected by July of that year, and 774 died.

Testing people with symptoms, isolating suspected cases, and restricting travel all likely contributed to the halt of the SARS epidemic. Curiously, data from seroepidemiologic studies conducted among food market workers in areas where the SARS epidemic presumably began showed that 40 percent of wild animal traders and 20 percent of individuals who worked with them were seropositive for SARS, meaning they had been exposed to the virus, although none had a history of having SARS-like illness. These findings suggest that many undiagnosed individuals were exposed through their occupation to a SARS-like virus. It also implies that exposure frequently caused asymptomatic infection (or infection subclinical enough to go unnoticed), yet this finding did not garner much attention as the outbreak was contained quickly.

The last series of documented cases of SARS to date have been laboratory-acquired, meaning from accidental exposure occurring in research labs working with the SARS-CoV.

The next major coronavirus outbreak, MERS, began in Saudi Arabia in 2012. Almost all of the nearly 2,500 cases affected people who lived in or traveled to the Middle East, thus the name source. A likely explanation for why this virus remained contained to the region was that this coronavirus was found to be less contagious than its SARS cousin. It was, however, much more deadly, killing 858 people while infecting far fewer than SARS. Although the number of deaths doesn't seem much higher than the 774 from SARS, the fatality rate, meaning the percentage of people who died based on the total number infected, was three times that of SARS (30 percent versus 10 percent).

The SARS and MERS outbreaks each burned out in less than a year and most people in the western hemisphere soon forgot about them. We have a short attention span when it comes to diseases that don't directly affect us. When cases of those diseases fell off, public health officials shifted to other emergencies such as Ebola and Zika, while coronavirus vaccine and treatment research funding dropped sharply. As a result, as most of us know all too well from experience, no successful vaccine existed for a coronavirus as we entered 2020.

While the greater scientific consensus since the beginning has been that a natural spillover from animals to humans created this novel virus, some also suggest the coronavirus causing the 2020 pandemic may be lab-manufactured. Others speculate that a lab accident may have leaked a natural virus housed in a controlled research laboratory into the human population. The sheer mention of such contrarian hypotheses can be considered xenophobic and offensive in some circles, but while we need to be careful to avoid biased conclusions, it is worth investigating the origins and cover-up of the virus in China.

We must be able to dispassionately consider the case at hand before coming to a decision about the truth, whatever it may be. So let's start with a manufactured virus: is this plausible? Could the virus have been bioengineered? To find the answer, let us begin with microbial engineering.

WHAT DOES AN ENGINEERED VIRUS LOOK LIKE?

Microbial engineering allows for the rapid production of viruses, bacteria, and other microbials, helping us address problems in everything from food production to public health. One of the most commonly used forms of microbial engineering is insulin production.

Insulin, taken directly from cattle and pigs, has been used for decades to treat the medical condition diabetes. Despite saving millions of lives, this animal-based insulin has also resulted in allergic reactions. To avoid the animal allergy, scientists created a synthetic version of human-based insulin in 1978 using the bacterium *E. coli*. Today, millions of diabetics worldwide use synthetic "human" insulin, made in both bacteria and yeast, to regulate their blood sugar levels.

Antiviral treatments and vaccine research also rely heavily on recombination techniques by growing viruses in various media, such as eggs, or in animal hosts.

When a vaccine is being produced, researchers will either "grow" the desired "target" virus in their labs or they will take a piece of the target virus and insert it into another virus known as the "vector" virus. The vector virus is typically a different type of virus altogether that is easily modified not to replicate in human cells. This process allows the body to form an immune response to the desired targeted virus without becoming clinically "infected" by the target or vector virus.

However, for a vaccine to be produced, there must be samples of the target virus available. Chemical synthesis of viral genomes provides a new and powerful tool for studying their pathogenic potential and developing possible treatments for it. This method is particularly useful if the natural viral template is not available. Thus, by experimenting with viruses, we can identify killer diseases before they appear in nature. At least, that's the idea.

Research that involves increasing a pathogen's transmissibility or virulence in order to study its potential is called "gain-of-function" research, and it has a history of ethical scrutiny. After a series of influenza-related lab accidents made headlines nearly a decade ago, the United States declared a moratorium on government financing for such research because of the risks posed by a possible lab accident causing an outbreak, as well as limited funding. The funding freeze, however, was short-lived, ending by 2017. At that time, the United States rejoined other countries, such as China, that did not have restrictions in place on gain-of-function research.

With improvements in genetic manipulation comes the need for additional tools to detect genetically modified pathogens that may occur in the environment, whether as developed for biological weaponry or accidental lab escapes, both having occurred throughout history.

Anthrax, a highly contagious disease caused by the bacterium *Bacillus anthracis*, carrying roughly a 90 percent fatality rate, can be created easily in a lab. It is incredibly durable, as the spores are able to lie dormant for years before reactivating and multiplying. This combination of characteristics makes anthrax a potentially dangerous bioterrorism weapon.

As such, anthrax has been used in warfare since World War I, when Germany sent infected animals to the Allies, and again during World War II by the British to weaken German livestock, resulting in famine.

More recently, in 2001, anthrax was used as a bioterrorism weapon in the United States, where envelopes with the pathogenic "white powder" spores were sent to politicians and various media outlets, resulting in five people dying.

Historically, when an act of bioterrorism occurs, it has been nearly impossible to link the pathogen back to its source. Following the 2001 anthrax attack, scientists were able to develop a method to trace anthrax spores to the local water supplies used in growing the spores. The technique measures minuscule quantities of the elements that exist in water from different parts of the United States (and world). While the method might not provide the precise location where the spores were grown, it potentially can narrow it down by region and even locality.

However, when it comes to evaluating viruses, the process is not as straightforward. The original SARS-CoV genome was found to be a mixture derived from multiple recombination events over time, as the virus made its way from bats to civets to humans, a common zoonosis pattern among Coronaviridae.

As the second week of January 2020 was coming to an end, the Chinese authorities finally shared the sequence of the new CoV genome they believed to be causing the emerging mystery illness, taken from patient samples in Wuhan. They, however, were less than accommodating in sharing virus samples for independent review and analysis.

Researchers pored over the preliminary published sequence attempting to identify where the virus came from. Often, when a genetic sequence is commercially synthesized, the scientists will leave a signature within it so they can differentiate the end product from a potential contaminate. It's like a tiny label that signals "man-made." Ohio State University researchers said there is "no credible evidence" of genetic engineering in a paper published in *Emerging Microbes & Infections*, following review of the provided genetic sequence.

Examination of the distributed genetic code by many other virologists plus independent reviews of succeeding patient samples have also not identified a manufactured signature or obvious break points in the genetic code that would verify synthetic splicing occurred. Naturally, molecular biologists reflexively report that there are no telltale signs of genetic manipulation in the circulating strains of SARS-CoV-2, indicating that a natural origin is likely.

The problem is, once the manufactured strain starts replicating, naturally occurring mutations can degrade the signatures, making them unrecognizable. In addition, while identifying available sequences using signatures helps detect and potentially discourage malicious genetic engineering purposes, there's no reason a genetic engineer *has* to include a signature. So an "unsigned" engineered pathogen could appear natural.

But there are other reasons to rule against the virus as a bioweapon or even as man-made. As virologist Robert F. Garry of Tulane University remarked, "The adaptations that the virus has made to affect humans are actually very different than what you would expect if you were designing it using computational models in biological engineering." In the same review, he proposed there was evidence for natural development because the SARS-CoV-2 spike protein was better at binding the human ACE2 cells and differing in mode of action than previously predicted. In addition, he explained, if someone was trying to engineer a new coronavirus as a pathogen, they would have added the mutations in the binding region to a backbone from an *existing* virus rather than creating a new one altogether.

However, as scientists have continued to report, the SARS-CoV-2 backbone differs substantially from known coronaviruses. Given all of this analysis, as well as the way the virus devastated Chinese cities, it's highly unlikely the virus was an engineered bioweapon intentionally released. But does that mean we have a good idea about where the virus actually came from? Not really, as the answer still means we have to rely on suspect Chinese information.

THE BAT CONNECTION

That the virus causing COVID-19 has something to do with bats has become common knowledge, but you may be surprised by how tenuous that connection is. We're essentially taking China's word for it. On January 23, 2020, Dr. Shi Zhengli of the Wuhan Institute of Virology (WIV) in Wuhan released a paper indicating that the new coronavirus was 96 percent identical to the ancestral bat strain coronavirus RaTG13, which her laboratory had isolated from Yun-nan (China) bats in 2013.

According to the paper, the lab collected bat feces and analyzed the samples for possible presence of coronaviruses. According to Dr. Shi, they only kept a record of the sequence and not the actual sample itself.

To put it into plainer words, *there is no physical proof for the existence of RaTG13 outside of WIV, and even then, they only report lab notes of it.*

For reasons unknown, they did not publish literature on the strain. This is curious, since the goal of the lab's research was to identify a coronavirus that has the potential to transfer to humans so they can work on treatments and vaccines, as well as keep a watchful eye on possible strains circulating in wildlife with human spillover potential. Yet, they did not print their findings on the strain until after the outbreak in 2020.

To this day, SARS-CoV-2 still shares the highest level of genetic similarity with RaTG13, after active investigations and sampling of bats worldwide. Still, RaTG13, as described in the Wuhan lab notes, is only 96 percent identical to SARS-CoV-2 and would have required further mutations to infect rodents and even more to spill over to humans.

Specifically, it's lacking a receptor-binding motif (RBM) region, the portion of the virus that encounters the host (animal or human) cell. Simply, RaTG13 cannot directly infect rodents or humans without a recombination event forming the RBM allowing it to recognize the different species.

In early 2020, other scientists in China identified a peculiar strain of the coronavirus from the rodent pangolin (pangolin-19). They found pangolin-19 to only be 90 percent similar to SARS-CoV-2, but the RBM region was nearly identical to it.

As the now famous Dr. Anthony Fauci, head of the National Institute of Allergy and Infectious Diseases, told *National Geographic* magazine, "Everything about the stepwise evolution over time strongly indicates that [this virus] evolved in nature and then jumped species."

The question is, how did a bat RNA virus evolve into a human pathogen that became widely contagious and deadly to humans? Articles in the press and in the scientific literature have endlessly examined scenarios by which this natural zoonotic transfer might have occurred.

Experts have universally seized upon the notion that the intermediate species was likely a pangolin given the near identical RBM region, allowing the mutation to develop, thereby enabling the virus to infect humans.

To this day, though, the novel virus has not been identified in the wild yet. Where and when did this happen? Why wasn't it discovered by scientists before it spilled over in the country with the largest coronavirus surveillance program in the world?

So, how did all of this transpire?

WET MARKETS

We've known about the dangers of wet markets for a while, so when one of the earliest reported cases of the mystery illness in China involved a patient who had recently been at a local wet market, no one should have been surprised.

Wet markets sell live poultry, fish, reptiles, and mammals of every kind. Some wet markets even sell wild or banned species like cobras, boars, dogs, and pangolins. Such markets are widespread predominantly in Asian countries and in areas where Asian people have migrated.

The infection danger lies in how crowded conditions allow viruses from different species to frequently swap genes because of close harboring quarters. As species stay in close proximity with one another in such a setting, virus mutation can easily occur. Live-poultry markets were identified as the source of the H5N1 avian "flu" virus that was transmitted to and killed people within Hong Kong. Because of this known phenomenon, researchers like those at WIV keep tabs on circulating viral strains in wildlife, especially in bats and those kept in the close quarters of wet markets. After civets were implicated to be the intermediate host for SARS in 2004, China banned wildlife in markets.

Still, on May 12, in a tweet on social media, the Chinese embassy said the seafood market in question did not sell bats at the time of the outbreak, while also denying the presence of "wildlife wet markets" to be present in China at all. While it is understandable bats may not have been listed on the inventory list of the wet market, it is well known that wet markets selling wildlife, sometimes illegal, such as civets and pangolins, are present within China, or at least, *were* at the time of the pandemic's origin. It was only in February 2020 that China banned the trade in and human consumption of wild animal life, as the country was then at the beginning of the outbreak.

As reported in *Nature*, pangolins were also not listed on the inventory of items being sold in Wuhan, but this omission could be deliberate since it would be illegal to have them there. The International Union for Conservation of Nature Species Survival Commission (SSC) Pangolin Specialist Group says pangolins are "the most illegally traded mammal in the world." It is not far-fetched to assume that illegal trafficking of pangolins was occurring even without documentation of it.

Two separate groups of virologists who analyzed the viral sequences say that the virus found in the pangolin is similar to the human version, with one saying the evolution to SARS-CoV-2 was possible and the other saying that it was unlikely. Such lack of consensus fuels alternative origin theories.

Garry and a team of Tulane University colleagues, examining the question of the natural evolution of SARS-CoV-2, determined it can be summed up by two scenarios:

"In one scenario," they wrote, "the virus evolved to its current pathogenic state through natural selection in a non-human host and then jumped to humans." This process occurred through cross-species recombination originating in bats, then jumping to an intermediate species where it gained the ability to move to humans through mutations, as SARS and MERS did. While the SARS and MERS originating strains have been found in their respective intermediate hosts (civets and dromedary camels), thus far, efforts to identify a similarly close link in the original pathway of SARS-CoV-2 into humans have failed.

The other scenario, according to Garry's team, is that "a non-pathogenic version of the virus [RaTG13] jumped from an animal host into humans and then evolved to its current pathogenic state within the human population" by a series of natural selection events within the human host. This would imply the virus became more infectious and dangerous as it circulated among humans, meaning it may have gone undetected in animals and humans prior to the current outbreak.

Either scenario may have happened. We still don't know and we may never know.

If only it stopped there.

A feature unique to SARS-CoV-2 is that the RBM spike protein has been found to be extremely efficient at binding to human cells. The presence of such similar optimal binding in the pangolin and human is theorized to be through convergent evolution (the virus's traits develop to adapt in differing environments), or an alternative possibility is that recombination events (in nature or a controlled setting) among different coronaviruses created the mutations and the "new" strain contains pieces of each virus in it.

In addition to the distinctive RBM mutation in the SARS-CoV-2 spike protein, another interesting piece to the spike protein that has scientists puzzled is that it has a unique furin cleavage site insertion.

FURIN SITE: THE KEY TO COVID-19'S SPREAD

While I did study and work in the immunology and microbiology arenas prior to medical school, I am certainly not an expert in the matter. But I will try to explain this in an understandable manner the best I can. The S "spike" protein has two main parts: the RBM that binds to the human cell that we already discussed and a second cleavage part that facilitates merging of the virus into the host cell. So, the RBM portion allows the virus to bind to the cell, while the cleavage portion incorporates the virus *into* the cell for replication and virulence. In other words, a virus really needs a furin-like cleavage site in order to replicate quickly in humans. Also, it seems the furin site in the novel coronavirus that is causing some of the most complex symptoms of the illness and contributing to its highly contagious nature.

Let's take a look at influenza, the virus that causes the flu every year. Each year the strains of influenza vary, which is why it is not only difficult to predict how bad the season will be but also warrants a new vaccine to be produced annually. When there is a highly pathogenic form of influenza, researchers have found it has a furin-like cleavage site that makes it more dangerous and contagious. Furin cleavage sites in other pathogens such MERS-CoV, anthrax, and RSV have also been shown to have higher pathogenicity.

While the particular furin cleavage site found in SARS-CoV-2 is not present in SARS-CoV or even RaGT13, it is suspected this mutation is what allowed SARS-CoV-2 to efficiently spread throughout the human population.

One constant with the illness caused by this novel virus has been that the elderly and those with chronic medical conditions have disproportionately been affected by the severity of the infection. Biotech entrepreneur Yuri Deigin suggested that "it is possible that the new furin site could also be largely responsible for the pronounced age-dependent morbidity and mortality of [SARS-]CoV2," as suggested in a study led by a University of Texas researcher:

Patients with hypertension, diabetes, coronary heart disease, cerebrovascular illness, chronic obstructive pulmonary disease, and kidney dysfunction have worse clinical outcomes when infected with SARS-CoV-2, for unknown reasons . . . Plasmin, and other proteases, may cleave a newly inserted furin site in the S protein of SARS-CoV-2, extracellularly, which increases its infectivity and virulence.

Patients with high blood pressure, renal disease, and other chronic illness have higher levels of circulating enzymes that interact with the furin site. The cleavage can result in a higher viral load, and can also increase inflammatory markers within the body, specifically D-dimer. Both higher viral loads and the presence of D-dimer are independent risk factors of disease severity and mortality with COVID-19. Also, D-dimer levels naturally increase with age, predisposing elderly patients to severe disease.

An interesting feature of COVID-19 is the presence of neurological symptoms, including loss of taste and smell.

In 2019, a group of scientists from various institutions in Beijing, including the China Agricultural University, demonstrated viral neurotropism (ability to affect the nervous system) using genetic engineering. The researchers manually inserted a furin cleavage site into a recombinant respiratory virus and infected a chicken with it, resulting in neurologic symptoms, demonstrating the ability to induce neurotropism.

Because of the known danger of furin site mutations, virologists have been studying them in coronaviruses for decades, and introducing artificial ones in labs. American scientists even inserted one *in vitro* while studying the first SARS-CoV in 2006.

Coincidentally, researchers at the Wuhan Institute of Virology, including the lead scientist, Shi Zhengli, have spent many years working on such projects, including inserting new furin sites into coronaviruses as well as interchanging the RBM of one virus with another.

At the end of October 2019, Ralph Baric, another well-known virologist, submitted for publication a paper on how spike protein protease cleavage (like a furin site) is important to crossing the "barrier to zoonotic infection" by coronaviruses.

By 2019, work involving altering the spike protein through furin and RBM manipulation was occurring at the Wuhan lab, thanks to a $3.7 million NIH grant titled *Understanding the Risk of Bat Coronavirus Emergence*. Shi Zhengli co-authored a paper supporting her mission and opinion calling for further research into synthetic viruses:

> **Currently, no clinical treatments or prevention strategies are available for any human coronavirus . . . Thus, future work should be focused on the biological properties of these viruses using virus isolation, reverse genetics and *in vitro* and *in vivo* infection assays.**

The Shi Zhengli group even published a paper in 2017 where they reported creating not one but eight synthetic viruses—all made using transplanted RBMs from bat SARS-like viruses.

Why do scientists create these killer viruses that have the potential to infect humans? The technical answer is that we need to understand the probability of natural zoonotic spillover outbreaks and to also develop treatments and vaccines should they occur in humans.

Scientists are tasked with identifying possible threats that may occur and discovering ways to either prevent them from happening or develop treatments to lessen their consequences. Undoubtedly, there are settings across the globe where wildlife and livestock live in close proximity to each other. As we see with humans, when a single member of the household falls ill, often, everyone else does because of the free swapping of air and exposure to surfaces, including restroom space. In animals, while one pathogen may not be able to directly infect another species initially, the continued repeated exposure allows the virus to eventually undergo mutations enabling it to infect other species.

Unfortunately, if scientists are unable to find the specific virus in nature, whether in bats or pangolins or another wildlife animal, it will be nearly impossible to definitively convince the masses that the virus had a natural origin.

To recap, we have a bat virus (RaTG13) that includes part of a pangolin virus (pangolin-19), which somehow acquired a "furin site" that allows it to bond with human cells. Thus far, there is no known common place for the bats containing the 96 percent genetically similar RaTG13 virus to come in contact with the pangolin-19 with the identical RBM to form SARS-CoV-2. Further, how the furin cleavage mutation developed also remains unknown.

So we have questions without answers.

There are very specific viral sequences that trace back to bats and pangolins in China consistent with some natural origin.

But there is less scientific data to calm suspicion that the virus, while it may have originated in nature, was being studied and possibly manipulated in a lab creating a chimera, as researchers are known to do. This brings up the possibility that the new recombinant virus "escaped" from a controlled laboratory setting.

A possibility is that the RaTG13 virus could have been injected into a pangolin for the purpose of studying potential virulence of this virus.

The process can occur by serial episodes of the rodent being exposed to the virus in a controlled manner, mimicking the natural zoonotic occurrences, a process that would be difficult to distinguish from a naturally occurring route.

If this were done, you would not expect to see the splice points in the genetic sequence or the signatures we discussed earlier.

So while it is conceivable that RaTG13 evolved in the pangolin providing the RBM, one very important piece of the novel SARS-CoV-2 is still missing from the genome: the genetic insertion that created a furin cleavage site unique to SARS-CoV-2.

While researchers focus on synthetic furin cleavage sites, it is crucial to note that through random mutations, coronaviruses can have many naturally occurring furin sites. The natural process of random mutation, Yuri Deigin writes, "is what happened in the case of MERS, as was pointed out in 2015 by an international team of authors, including Shi Zhengli and Ralph Baric."

So, did RaTG13 cross over in pangolins to form the novel pathogen? Maybe, but it would have required two separate recombination events to turn itself into the virus that is circulating around the globe today. All of this is certainly feasible in nature—after all, these viruses mutate and recombine constantly.

Yet, some virologists remain puzzled. Where did this genetic insert come from? The most genetically similar bat CoV RaTG13 does not have the specific furin cleavage site. The pangolin-19 doesn't either. Neither do any other known coronaviruses. While it is possible that it was manually inserted using genetic engineering through gain-of-function research, it is also possible another natural recombination event occurred naturally with a yet-to-be-found coronavirus in nature.

If the experts are puzzled, imagine how the rest of us feel.

What we do know is that the cleavage of RBM and furin subunits of the spike protein creates efficient binding to human ACE2 by SARS-CoV-2, allowing it to proficiently infect and be transmitted among humans, causing the global COVID-19 pandemic.

DID HISTORY REPEAT ITSELF?

The 1977–1978 influenza epidemic is another outbreak that some scientists believe may not have occurred naturally. Martin Furmanski, a medical doctor who works for an antinuclear nonprofit, claims the H1N1 influenza virus *may have* accidentally been released by a laboratory in Russia while developing a flu vaccine. He cites a 1978 paper which noted that the contemporary influenza virus was the same as a virus from 1950. The outbreak turned into a global pandemic that spread fear across the globe. The pandemic did not cause the devastation that is occurring with COVID-19, as in that case historic immunity from prior exposure to the virus resulted in fewer deaths. Furmanski in an article for the Center for Arms Control and Nonproliferation, continued:

> Only since 2009–2010 did major papers begin to state directly the 1977 emergence of H1N1 influenza was a laboratory related release . . . The most plausible reason for a Chinese or Russian laboratory to thaw out and begin growing a c1950 H1N1 virus in 1976–77 was as a response to the US 1976 "swine flu" program, which resulted in a program to immunize the entire US population against H1N1 influenza virus . . . Thawing available frozen stocks of virus was necessary, because H1N1 was no longer circulating. Modern commentators have begun to articulate this connection between the 1976 swine flu immunization program and the 1977 H1N1 re-emergence.

Scientists and researchers have warned that experiments with virulent pathogens, such as smallpox, Ebola, and various influenza viruses, are inherently dangerous, requiring oversight and strict regulation, which is why they require severe laboratory compliance. Yet, since the quelling of the original SARS outbreak in 2003, there have been six documented SARS-CoV outbreaks originating from research laboratories, including four in China.

Could a processing error or a safety mishap have caused the COVID-19 pandemic? Sure—it has happened before. Yuri Deigin argues:

> Several options are possible—from a leak during development of a potential vaccine to fundamental research on laboratory recombination of the bat and pangolin viruses. Some particularly ambitious researcher could even decide to combine the two "fashionable research themes"—adding a furin site and

transplanting RBM from a strain of one species (pangolin) to another (bats), so that later, confirming the increased virulence of the new chimeric virus, they can wax poetic about the dangers of the same recombination happening in Yunnan caves or wet markets.

It's all possible. However, possibilities do *not* prove that the evolution of SARS-CoV-2 involved microbial engineering. They don't disprove it either.

WUHAN INSTITUTE OF VIROLOGY

One troubling coincidence that cannot be ignored is that the initial outbreak of the novel virus occurred in the city of Wuhan, which happens to frequently publish on bat coronavirus research. The wet market where the outbreak was suspected to occur was less than ten miles from the only lab in the world containing the virus most genetically similar to the one causing the current pandemic, the Wuhan Institute of Virology.

Indeed, no one other than the Wuhan lab has ever seen RaTG13. And RaTG13 is a very unusual strain, per their reports. It is also odd that Shi Zhengli's group was silent about the strain for all these years since it is quite different from its SARS-like siblings, especially in its spike protein, which is precisely the component that determines which type of host this virus can infect.

Given how close the Wuhan lab and the wet market are to each other, many, including researchers and news sources like *The Washington Post* and *Newsweek*, have postulated that an accidental leak from the lab is a strong possibility. The speculation is that one of the two labs in Wuhan working with coronaviruses could have accidentally let a virus obtained from nature escape, or that the lab was genetically modifying a virus that then escaped.

Yuri Deigin writes that "giving credence to the lab hypothesis, there are reports that in 2018, American experts were quite alarmed after their visit to the Wuhan Institute of Virology."

The Washington Post reported that people who had seen and were familiar with the inspection reports, known as "cables," said they raised concerns about the safety protocols at the Wuhan Institute of Virology lab:

> **"During interactions with scientists at the WIV laboratory, they noted the new lab has a serious shortage of appropriately trained technicians and investigators needed to safely operate this high-containment laboratory," states the Jan. 19, 2018, cable, which was drafted by two officials from the embassy's environment, science and health sections who met with the WIV scientists. (The State Department declined to comment on this and other details of the story.)**

Columnist Josh Rogin of *The Washington Post* obtained one leaked cable that specifically highlights alarms that its work on bat coronaviruses could be unsafe. Xiao Qiang, a research scientist at the University of California at Berkeley, said: "The cable tells us that there have long been concerns about the possibility of the threat to public health that came from this lab's research, if it was not being adequately conducted and protected."

This may sound alarming, but cables demonstrating lab safety issues, although they make for a good headline during a global pandemic, can be misleading. They certainly are not the smoking gun that many want them to be. The truth is, such cables are written by political officers and interpreted by political science graduates. Investigations by hierarchal organizations, like The Joint Commission in the U.S. hospital system, are meant to find faults and errors, regardless of how minor or clinically insignificant they may be. Think of the dramatization of a home inspection report upon selling a home. The way the report is written would make you believe the house is a hazard to anyone who steps foot in it.

While the cables highlight the potential for safety hazards to exist, they don't prove such hazards resulted in a leak.

Further material that fueled conspiracy theorists, albeit of the sort that is difficult to confirm, was information obtained by the London-based NBC News Verification Unit that indicates there was limited cellphone activity in a high-security portion of the Wuhan Institute of Virology in mid-October. The lack of activity prompted questions as to whether an event occurred that required the lab to decrease activity at the time.

The information was gathered from commercially available cellphone location data, which noted a decrease in lab activity in early October, while traffic studies also showed travel to the lab remained light for the next month.

United States intelligence agencies also received cellphone and satellite data suggesting decreased activity at the lab, indicating a possible shutdown. However, after examining their own data, the U.S. agencies were unable to confirm such a shutdown occurred, deeming the reports to be "inconclusive."

Even the most secure laboratories have accidents. The larger point to keep in mind is that the presence of biological research leaves open a range of plausible explanations. And with that, opinions.

While conducting research for this book, I reached out to an old colleague and friend who has spent much of her professional career researching Coronaviridae, to understand better the plausibility of a natural origin based on the genetic sequence of this virus. After I sent the email with my questions and a link to a scientific opinion article, I received a response essentially saying she would not engage in a conversation that promulgates conspiracy theories regarding the viral origin. This was a glimpse into the notion that questioning the popular opinion, that the virus had a natural origin with environmental zoonotic spillover, was anti-science, and basically a conspiracy theory.

In reality, I was seeking science-based information from a trusted coronavirus virologist to shed light upon and potentially dispel the lab-born theories and help me understand what could have happened. My reason for wanting to connect was because such theories circulating were causing angst in people who were feeling sabotaged by a foreign adversary, therefore hindering their ability to move forward in a productive manner. However, rather than being given the opportunity to engage in an intelligent discussion, I was disregarded—canceled.

As I wrote in the introduction, experts are in a unique position to explain why conspiracy theories are wrong, but if they refuse to answer questions, it doesn't help the cause of science. We need to have these conversations. If experts don't speak to these issues, people will turn to conspiracists. Sadly, what has occurred within the United States is that people are designated as being anti-science, or even promoting Sinophobia, if they question information from China and the natural spillover theory.

The early lack of transparency and delays give credence to those suspecting China has something to hide.

The question is: what?

A vital clue as to the origin of SARS-CoV-2 could be determined by a seroprevalence study of inspecting blood samples from various places around China that had been stored prior to January 2020 to see if there were circulating antibodies in populations indicating earlier exposure and localizing the region of origin. This would give credence to the natural selection theory mentioned earlier.

If there is no information available of prior community exposure and the virus cannot be identified in the wild, then a thorough investigation of the WIV and its bat coronavirus research should be allowed. An independent investigation of the facility is likely to be the only way to refute theories of a lab escape, yet the heightened geopolitical climate is unlikely to allow such efforts and at this point, evidence is probably lost. It wasn't until February 2021, over a year later, and with evidence gone, that the CCP finally allowed the World Health Organization to investigate the wet market.

Deep inquiries should be made about the overarching wisdom of removing viruses from the wild and performing "what-if" gain-of-function research on them, given the long, well-documented global history of lab mistakes and leaks.

The questioning of the viral origin was only the tip of the iceberg when it came to the anti-science accusations that followed the virus across the world.

The truth is, we don't *know* what happened yet. We don't know for certain where the virus originated or how it evolved to become a human pathogen. Today, there is still no definitive evidence to prove or disprove much of the theories, and it is dangerously divisive to dismiss people as *anti-science* who still have questions. While the natural spillover of the virus remains the most probable theory, it is not outlandish to question the proximity of the coronavirus research lab to the outbreak site and whether or not it played a role. For now, there are probabilities and a few strange coincidences—but coincidence is not proof. And ultimately, the origin has little significance at this point.

CHAPTER 10

THE CHINESE COVER-UP BEGINS

How could they see anything but the shadows if they were never allowed to move their heads?

—PLATO, *THE ALLEGORY OF THE CAVE*

In the United States, we tend to name airports after individuals who have acquired renown. When we leave Washington, D.C., for example, we do so via Ronald Reagan Washington National Airport or, if we are willing to put up with the drive, Dulles International, which is named after former Secretary of State John Foster Dulles. But in China, there is much more reluctance about singling out individuals—other than Mao Zedong, the former chair of the Chinese Communist Party (CCP), or his successor, Xi Jinping—for honorific purposes.

Chinese airports tend to be named after cities or districts of cities. Thus, the airport in Hong Kong is simply Hong Kong International Airport. Designed by British architectural firm Foster + Partners and completed in 1998, the airport has been described in lyrical terms by architectural critics. According to an article in *The Guardian*, "From above, the roof gives the building the appearance not of the sea serpent seen from road, train or ferry, but of an aircraft on a scale that not even Howard Hughes would have dreamt of."

On April 28, 2020, a woman made her way within this huge edifice toward a specific destination: Level 7 of Terminal 1. She was on her way to catch a Cathay Pacific flight to the United States.

Most of us have gone through the necessary hassle and anxiety of preparing for a flight. Dr. Li-Meng Yan had a different reason for worrying about whether she would make it onto the plane. Yan, a postdoctoral virology researcher at the Hong Kong School of Public Health, was carrying what she believed to be dangerous baggage in the form of what she herself, following her arrival in the United States, would call "the message of the truth of COVID."

The 26-page document of "truth" that Dr. Yan sought to convey contained allegations that China would not want to get out: that concealment had occurred and was still occurring regarding COVID-19. This was not a truth that could be told in Hong Kong, considering the historic censorship of negative press. If she had told it in that context, she stated, she would have been "disappeared and killed."

While the report pushed by Dr. Yan was not peer reviewed and thus open to scrutiny from fellow researchers, it fell in line with a hallmark of the pandemic: the rapid influx of freely shared information to hasten the process of discovery. The practice of posting "preprints," data that hasn't undergone formal review, does have its advantages; it is also easily disregarded as anti-science.

When she arrived in the United States, Yan found that few people wanted to hear her testimony. True, she appeared in a featured segment on Fox News, but almost no attention was paid to her beyond that. The problem with ignoring contrarian thought, whether it is validated or not, is that the public censoring of individuals grabs hold of vulnerable people and breeds distrust.

The censoring of this individual was an example of how the mainstream media minimized China's culpability in the virus's origin and spread. As China silenced dissent and covered up the facts, our media and elites admonished President Trump for calling COVID-19 the "Chinese virus." CNN and Yale School of Medicine called that term "inaccurate." They also complained that it was "stigmatizing" and "xenophobic," which is up for debate—since I can name more pathogens named after their region of origin than not. It's no wonder liberal journalists ignored Yan's story: it went against the narrative that America was the worst villain in the COVID crisis—more specifically, President Trump was the villain. Once again, people were letting politics interfere with the process of fact gathering.

Once Yan appeared on Fox, other media outlets steered clear of her. On social media, she was pilloried. One post on Twitter read as follows:

> shes so disgusting. 8 wuhan whistleblowers except for dr li wenliang tragedically died of covid19 all live well in wuhan today while she said gov would kill her? did she provide any hard scientific evidence as a doctor? shes just a liar leaving her husband to get a green card

The writer must have assumed that none of those reading this tweet would take the time to do any research and to find out that, in fact, Wuhan whistleblowers and citizen journalists Chen Qiushi, Fang Bin, and Li Xehua (to name only a few of which we are aware) are still very much missing at the time of this writing. And prominent whistleblowers who have resumed their pre-pandemic roles may be subject to CCP pressure and unable to speak candidly.

Beijing-based millionaire Ren Zhiqiang, who harshly criticized the CCP response to SARS-CoV-2, was detained in March 2020 and spent months awaiting criminal charges. The CCP also suspended his membership and shut down his Weibo account (China's version of Twitter), on which at the time he had over 37 million followers. Another critic, distinguished law professor and jurist Xu Zhangrun, was detained in July 2020 and later released.

In an essay entitled "Viral Alarm: When Fury Overcomes Fear," published before his detention, Zhangrun spoke sharply and clearly about the harm that CCP officials had done to the Chinese people:

The authorities proved themselves to be at a loss as to how to respond effectively, and the high cost of their impotence was soon visited upon the common people. Before long, the coronavirus was reaching around the globe and the People's Republic found itself rapidly isolated from the rest of the world. It was as though the China famed for its "Reform and Opening-Up" policies for more than three decades was being undone in front of our very eyes. In one fell swoop, it seemed as though the People's Republic, and in particular its vaunted system of governance, had been cast back to pre-modern times. As word spread about blockades being thrown up by towns and cities in an attempt to seal themselves against contagion, as doors were slammed shut everywhere, it actually felt as though we were being overwhelmed by the kind of primitive panic more readily associated with the Middle Ages.

Conspiracy theories aside, the world needs transparency from the Chinese. An open dialogue of information would have helped us to understand exactly how this started so contact tracing could begin, ultimately resulting in less spread and lives saved. Complete transparency would also have potentially dispelled the tidal wave of blame coming China's way.

In Plato's *Allegory of the Cave*, people who had always lived in a cave mistook shadows on a wall for reality. They were actually images created by puppet-masters standing outside with a light. The narrative advanced by the Chinese government is so different from the global scientific consensus that it's like the shadows on the wall projected toward prisoners in the allegory. The prisoners in the cave were wrongfully led to believe a perceived truth; however, once they turned around they noticed the shadows were an illusion caused by manipulators of reality lurking behind them.

Today, it remains unclear what occurred during the early days of the outbreak. The possibility of an apolitical investigation is dwindling—not just because of COVID fatigue but because so many details have been fabricated and much evidence destroyed. Would the outcome have changed had initial actions been different? If so, did mishandling occur because the world was fixated on the shadows on the wall while the Chinese Communist Party manipulated the elements behind us?

Transparency is central to understanding what occurred and how to move forward. However, notorious for its obstructionist response to external inquiry, China has impeded such investigations into their early handling of the crisis.

China failed to prepare for the crisis, ignoring warning signs from prior epidemics. When the crisis began, doctors were so tangled in red tape that they couldn't share information effectively. Since the Chinese Communist Party did not want to admit culpability, it obscured the origins of the outbreak, silencing whistleblowers and scrubbed away evidence. It was only through the bravery of those leaking the truth about COVID-19, and the conscientiousness of nations who put the pieces together, that the free world realized a deadly pandemic was on our doorsteps. China blithely concealed SARS-CoV-2's true danger, allowing it to spread unchecked throughout the world. This is the most anti-science you can be.

FAILED PREPAREDNESS

The thing is, China had plenty of warning that this crisis was coming. Following the 2003 SARS-CoV outbreak, Chinese public health officials put in place a robust surveillance system to monitor for any future outbreaks, a centralized system in which hospitals could easily input patient data alerting government officials of a brewing outbreak. Beijing could then monitor hospitals throughout the territories, assessing for trends that might go unseen by local officials and attempting to contain an outbreak before it spread.

While doctors in Wuhan began treating dozens of patients with the mystery illness in late 2019, rather than inputting the information into the system, hospitals deferred to local health officials.

Once Beijing became aware of the evolving situation, local officials set narrow criteria for testing and positive case reporting which had to be confirmed by bureaucrats before being officially recorded. Hospitals were also ordered to include only patients with direct connections to the wet market.

RESTRICTIONS. ADMINISTRATIVE BLOAT. SILENCE.

As accounts tell of people lining up outside the hospitals in Wuhan, the Chinese government remained quiet on the spreading contagion. Experts say that had the Chinese been more transparent, even a few days earlier, the course of the pandemic might have been greatly altered, with drastically less severe global consequences.

HUMAN LIFE. ECONOMIC RUIN. SOCIETIES IN PERIL.

The magnitude of their silence will perhaps one day be recounted, ideally told strictly with reference to empirical and research-proven facts.

As mentioned earlier, when people lack certain information, they turn to opinion, which is often informed by rumor more than fact. This is where we are now. In such a climate, we are forced to rely on scientists and medical professionals claiming to have access to truth.

Such experts, though, do not live in outer space, but rather in the midst of settings in which fear, danger, and power play crucial roles in influencing decision-making and actions.

For now, when it comes to the early days of the pandemic in China, what we have is the slippery territory of human beings recounting their truths about what happened that do *not* match what their government was portraying, and can never be made to match up.

Good science takes time. The unsettled and still evolving debate between competing theories regarding the course of the pandemic will continue to move down two tracks: the slow, laborious pathway of scientific and statistical research conducted in universities, academic teaching hospitals, corporations, and other institutions, and the fast track of trial and error, rumor, and popular opinion as conveyed through social media, whistleblowers, and other means.

The slow track assumes, as a starting point, that we can reasonably distinguish between unreliable sources and indisputable data, between opinion and provable facts, and, ultimately, between lies and truth. In contrast, the fast-track debate tends to blur distinctions for the sake of attracting attention, gaining professional status, and potentially putting forth one's own narrative.

I should stress the fact that, as a physician, I don't care where the virus came from. *However, it is my opinion that we must examine the consequences that a less-than-forthcoming China has had on the COVID debate before we can move forward as a global society working together to recover and rebuild.*

With all due caution regarding the very real threat of Sinophobia and the politicization of science, it is difficult to avoid thinking about SARS-CoV-2 at least partly in terms of the human drama between nations.

The stalemate between Chinese officials and the rest of the world has led to a global epistemological crisis that if not dealt with could wreak cataclysmic damage. As a May 26, 2020, article in *The Wall Street Journal* notes, according to the Pew Research Center, "84% of Americans said they distrust information from China's government about the outbreak, with 49% indicating zero trust in that information."

FINDING PATIENT ZERO

Patient zero has yet to be identified in the SARS-CoV-2 outbreak.

Although most reports indicate the earliest cases were found in

December 2019, the Chinese Communist Party may have known about the outbreak even earlier. According to government data seen by the *South China Morning Post* (*SCMP*), a 55-year-old man from Hubei province could have been the first person to have contracted the viral illness in mid-November. Unfortunately, no further information about this claim has become available.

However, we do know, as reported by *The Wall Street Journal* (*WSJ*), that on December 16 a 65-year-old man was admitted to Wuhan Central Hospital with fever and pneumonia. According to a report compiled by the House Foreign Affairs Committee Minority Staff, "He was treated with antibiotics and anti-flu medication, but his condition did not improve. It would later be discovered that he worked at the Huanan Seafood Wholesale Market." He was not the only hospitalized patient across the city with a similar presentation.

Exponential growth began. The SCMP reported the first double-digit daily rise in suspected "mystery illness" cases that same week, with over 30 patients in the hospital with comparable symptoms. By December 20, the number of cases doubled to 60 people, with the *WSJ* reporting the growing cases included family members in close contact with the wet market worker, but who had not gone to the market themselves.

An important thing to note: *This was an early sign of human-to-human transmission.*

As Christians across the world woke up on December 25 to celebrate Christmas, medical staff at two different hospitals in Wuhan were being quarantined after contracting the illness themselves.

This was a second indication human-to-human transmission was occurring.

Doctors were starting to warn officials that something unusual was happening. On December 27, Zhang Jixian, a doctor from Hubei Provincial Hospital of Integrated Chinese and Western Medicine, told China's health authorities (including the local branch of the Chinese Center for Disease Control and Prevention) that "the disease was being caused by a new strain of coronavirus that was 87%

genetically similar to SARS-CoV, the virus that caused the 2003 SARS pandemic."

Xinhua Net later reported:

Zhang's experience during the 2003 SARS outbreak, when she worked as a medical expert investigating suspected patients in Wuhan, made her sensitive to signs of an epidemic. After reading the CT images of the elderly couple, she summoned their son, demanding a CT scan of him too.

"At first their son refused to be examined. He showed no symptoms or discomfort, and believed we were trying to cheat money out of him," said Zhang. It was Zhang's insistence that brought her the second piece of evidence: the son's lungs showed the same abnormities as those of his parents.

"It is unlikely that all three members of a family caught the same disease at the same time unless it is an infectious disease," Zhang told Xinhua.

Also on Dec. 27, the hospital received another patient who also developed symptoms of coughing and fever and showed the same lung findings on the CT scan.

Suspecting an unknown, transmissible respiratory illness and filing the report, Zhang cordoned off an area in the department's ward to hospitalize the family. She then demanded that medics in the ward use enhanced personal protective equipment (PPE), anticipating the contagiousness of the illness.

Xinhua News wrote, "The arrivals of another three patients with similar lung issues in the next two days further alarmed the hospital, which on Dec. 29 convened a panel of 10 experts to discuss the seven cases. Their conclusion that the situation was extraordinary prompted the hospital to report directly to the municipal and provincial health authorities. Upon receiving the report, the authorities on the same day ordered an epidemiological investigation. That evening, experts from Wuhan Jinyintan Hospital, a hospital designated to treat contagious diseases, visited Zhang's hospital and fetched all but one of the patients.

The alarm was being raised elsewhere as well. Several days later, on December 30, Dr. Ai Fen, a physician who ran the emergency department at another hospital, Wuhan Central, received the results of a laboratory test for a patient identifying the cause of the illness to be a "SARS coronavirus." She then alerted her hospital administrative supervisors and reported the results to the Department of Public Health.

Ai would go on to tell *People* magazine (in an interview that was later censored) that tests showed a patient at her hospital came in in mid-December with an unknown coronavirus infection. In later media interviews, Ai said that China's censorship delayed the adoption of appropriate safety measures against the contagious illness, which ultimately contributed to its spread.

By the end of December, there were reports of over 180 people having been infected. Still, the alarm from the central surveillance system had not yet been sounded.

Meanwhile, red tape prevented doctors from testing samples and testing for the virus more widely. Although doctors in Wuhan had been collecting specimens from suspected cases in December, some were unable to confirm their findings because they were bogged down by having to get approval from the Chinese CDC. Medical personnel were ordered not to disclose any information about the new disease to the public and were told tests couldn't be run on patients who were not connected with the wet market. Chinese officials were circling the wagons and hiding information about what would turn out to be a global pandemic.

By then, the concept of human-to-human transmission of an unknown pathogen was cinched. While the local authorities weren't ready to announce an outbreak, a young doctor at a neighboring hospital did.

It was with his actions that word leaked out. After hours on December 30, Dr. Li Wenliang, an ophthalmologist at Wuhan Central

Hospital, armed with a photo of laboratory test results, sounded the alarm about the mystery illness for the first time with colleagues in a private discussion group on the Chinese messaging service WeChat. Immediately, his messages were shared widely on the microblogging website Weibo and the word of a possible contagious outbreak was out.

However, the messages weren't limited to health care professionals; they were also seen by the public and, more importantly, governmental officials. Only 48 hours later, on January 1, 2020, Li and several other doctors were brought in by CCP authorities to be questioned. Following several hours of interrogation, Li was released after signing a statement recognizing that he had "spread false rumors." Later, Li publicly shared the paperwork he had received from the police, which said, "We hope you can calm down and reflect on your behavior." A few weeks later, Li developed a fever and cough and was subsequently hospitalized after treating a patient for glaucoma who unknowingly also had the mystery illness.

After testing positive himself for the virus on February 1, the 34-year-old Dr. Li Wenliang tragically died only six days later, leaving behind a pregnant wife and young son.

SMALL BUT MIGHTY TAIWAN ALERTED THE WORLD TO THE VIRUS

Such leaks and whistleblowers were essential to the sharing of information early in the pandemic. The day after Li Wenliang shared the photo of lab results, another leak alerted the Taiwanese of the virus. Unofficial Chinese media reports began circulating toward the end of December of an "atypical pneumonia" outbreak, and a machine translation of one such report was posted December 31 on an American information-sharing platform.

Later that same day after seeing the information, an official from the Taiwan Centers for Disease Control sent an email to the World

Health Organization focal point, informing them of online reports concerning "at least seven atypical pneumonia cases" in Wuhan.

In the email, the Taiwanese official relayed that sick patients were supposedly being separated from the rest of the hospital population, in isolation, indicating there was suspected human-to-human spread of the virus. The WHO responded via a statement saying the concerns expressed were being forwarded to appropriate personnel but would not be posted publicly for others to see.

WHO headquarters in Geneva instructed the WHO China Country Office to try to verify these reports with the People's Republic of China (PRC) government.

By contrast, Taiwan's government believed the evidence of human-to-human transmission to be so great that on the same day they contacted the WHO, the Taiwanese instituted enhanced border control and quarantine measures "based on the assumption that human-to-human transmission was in fact occurring."

SINGAPORE

The response in Singapore was also quick and efficient. The country had good reason to be cautious. The SARS outbreak in 2003 caused Singapore's economy to suffer billions of dollars in losses and a rise in unemployment. Still recovering from the negative effects of the prior outbreak, the government was hell-bent not to have a repeat this time around. Rather than following the lead of the WHO and the CCP, they swiftly acted.

On January 2, 2020, days after the first public report of the disease from China, the Ministry of Health in Singapore developed a local case definition for the illness and mandated all suspected cases undergo nasal swab testing with results reporting to a centralized system. They also instituted screening protocols of travelers, contact tracing, and public campaign messages encouraging increased hand hygiene. Even asymptomatic contacts were put under quarantine in an attempt to halt transmission of the virus. While there was a potential for this inconvenience to be unnecessary, the price of proactive discipline is often less than the pain of regret, a pain that Singapore had suffered before when depending on the CCP for public health guidance.

At the time, Taiwan and Singapore were criticized for overreacting, but they were right. As of late March, 2021, Taiwan has had ten COVID deaths out of 969 cases and Singapore has had 29 deaths after 60,033 cases. That's not just for the month. That's for the *entire pandemic by that point.*

These were countries that learned their historical lessons well. Their pandemic preparation started back in 2004, after the last SARS epidemic, and they didn't let up in their efforts.

Even when there were only a very few cases reported in China, Taiwanese health authorities were already going onto each flight coming from Wuhan checking people for symptoms.

While the world looked upon these actions as alarmist, countries adjacent to China were acting on lessons learned the hard way. Because of SARS, they already had experience in dealing with a less-than-forthcoming mainland China, so they did not take any chances and put credence in the unofficial stories of what was occurring.

DESTRUCTION OF EVIDENCE

Back in China, the cover-up was underway. Local reports recount that in late December there were workers in protective gear cleaning the Huanan Seafood Wholesale Market in Wuhan, the wet market linked early to several cases of the mystery illness. According to witnesses, the workers were going stall-to-stall spraying disinfectant throughout the market before a public statement about the potential outbreak had even been made.

In November 2020, *The New York Times* discovered contrary

accounts regarding what occurred when Chinese CDC officials visited the wildlife market to investigate the virus's origin a few days after the market was cleaned. One official account reported that experts took samples from the animals sold there as well as other sources such as door handles and surfaces. George F. Gao, the chief scientist at China's CDC, told a reporter by the time his team arrived at the market it had been closed and sanitized, and that they were therefore unable to conduct a thorough investigation for a potential animal source of origin.

As *The New York Times* reported:

> The discrepancy in the accounts leaves open two possibilities. If researchers tested samples from live animals, then they may be concealing potentially important clues about the origins of the virus.
>
> But if they arrived after the market had been closed and disinfected, they may only have taken samples from places like door handles, counters and sewage runoff. Many outside experts consider this the most likely scenario. They said it was understandable that local officials, focused on preventing human illness, would rush to clean the market rather than pause to preserve evidence.
>
> Yet that would mean that Chinese officials probably missed a chance to confirm where the outbreak did, or did not, originate.

Understandably, the need to control a spreading pathogen by sanitizing seems prudent, but containment, investigation, *then* sanitization is how science works. Cloak-and-dagger operations hidden from the public eye that destroy the very evidence necessary to tackle the problem call into question the CCP's true intentions. The basic fact that they said samples were taken prior to destruction, followed by clarifications that the samples were actually destroyed, is equivalent to scientific blasphemy. Quietly trying to control a problem while keeping the public in the dark and providing little information to scientists is cutting public health efforts off at the knees.

The cover-up continued. A few days after the covert sanitation of the market, on January 3, the National Health Commission issued a nationwide order requiring that all samples of the virus be destroyed. By that point scientists at the Wuhan Institute of Virology had completed genetic mapping of the novel virus obtained from patient samples, but they had not publicly published the data or supplied it to the World Health Organization.

The CCP refused to acknowledge that they'd issued the destruction-of-evidence order until May 15, 2020, when the National Health Commission's Liu Dengfeng told reporters that they had "decided to temporarily manage the pathogen causing the pneumonia as Class II—highly pathogenic—and . . . destroy[ed] the samples."

The WHO did not even make public its knowledge of the outbreak in Wuhan until January 4, the day after the samples had been destroyed, when it issued a tweet:

> #China Has Reported to WHO a Cluster of #Pneumonia Cases -with No Deaths- in Wuhan, Hubei Province. Investigations Are Underway to Identify the Cause of This Illness.

Also that day, Dr. Ho Pak-Leung, the head of the University of Hong Kong's Centre for Infection, warned human-to-human transmission was highly possible, as reported by journalist Jimmy Choi in RTHK. Dr. Ho stated, according to the congressional report, that "he believed it was already occurring in Wuhan, due to the rapid increase in reported cases, and warned about a potential surge of cases" in the upcoming travel season.

Professor Zhang Yongzhen, a public health researcher in Shanghai, informed China's National Health Commission on January 5 that his team had been able to sequence the genome of the virus and that it resembled the SARS coronavirus from 2003.

"For a second time," the congressional report on COVID-19 origins explained, "the CCP failed to notify the WHO that Chinese researchers had identified the virus, sequenced its genome, and that it was a coronavirus genetically similar to the virus responsible for the 2003 SARS pandemic."

During the same week of January, the United States Centers for Disease Control and Prevention repeatedly contacted Chinese officials, offering to send a team of experts to assist with their response and begin their own independent investigation. The CCP reportedly declined to allow the U.S. teams to enter the People's Republic of China.

On January 8, *The Wall Street Journal* let the cat out of the bag and reported that the outbreak was being caused by a novel coronavirus. The congressional report lays out what happened next:

> Two days later, the CCP publicly acknowledged the novel coronavirus as the cause of the outbreak, but claimed "there is no evidence that the new virus is readily spread by humans, which would make it particularly dangerous, and it has not been tied to any deaths." This announcement was 13 days after Wuhan hospital officials informed CCP health authorities the virus responsible for the outbreak was a coronavirus genetically similar to SARS-CoV . . .

Frustrated that the CCP had not taken action in response to his January 5 warning, Shanghai Public Health Clinical Centre's Professor Zhang Yongzhen published his lab's genomic sequencing data of SARS-CoV-2 on virological.org and GenBank, an open access online database maintained by the National Center for Biotechnology Information within the U.S. National Institutes of Health. Hours later, the CCP's National Health Commission announced that it would provide the WHO with the virus's genomic sequencing. They also cracked down on the whistleblower lab, for the following day, January 12, the CCP, according to a February 28, 2020, article in the *South China Morning Post*, closed the Shanghai lab for "rectification."

Meanwhile, the Wuhan Institute of Virology published online its own viral genomic sequence that it had finalized ten days prior.

A couple of questions come to mind here: Why wasn't the Shanghai lab's sequence allowed to be submitted to the WHO? The WIV reports they had the sequence available ten days before it was publicly released—why was there a delay? If they hadn't completed it or they weren't confident in their data, why was it ordered for *all* viral samples to be destroyed, leaving them without samples to study in order to make tests, treatments, and a potential vaccine? Further, once the sequencing was completed by WIV, the virologists who did so must have known that they were dealing with a novel, highly virulent, and contagious coronavirus. Why didn't they sound the alarm?

It seems that Shanghai lab professor Zhang's online publication is what forced the CCP to finally share the genetic sequence with the world. While the sequence was eventually provided, by destroying the viral samples, they eliminated any external dispute and independent investigation.

Imagine if this information had been provided ten days earlier, before the beginning of the largest international travel season of the year. How many lives would have been saved?

Days later, the first death related to the outbreak was reported in Chinese state media on January 11, as travelers from across China began to depart for the annual Spring Festival travel season.

THE VIRUS GOES HOME FOR THE HOLIDAYS

Every year, the highlight of the national calendar in China is the New Year, also known as the time of the Spring Festival. The travel season for this special time of year lasts 40 days. It marks the renewal of the year, and the victory of the forces of life over those that threaten death. But in 2020, festive public gatherings, as well as holiday-related travel, created conditions under which the deadly, unseen virus could spread rapidly.

The Spring Festival season lasts approximately from January 10 to February 18, and during this time almost all of China moves. Indeed, the Lunar New Year is the time of the largest human migration on earth. China's elaborate railway system faces an extremely high traffic load and as described in an article by Maggie Hiufu Wong posted on the CNN website on January 10, 2020, experts estimate approximately 3 billion domestic and international trips occur in conjunction with the holiday.

The virus spread beyond China. On January 13, days after the genomic sequence was transmitted to the WHO, the first case of the illness, now referred to as Coronavirus Disease 2019 (COVID-19), outside of the PRC was reported in Thailand.

Still, China and the WHO denied confirmation of human-to-human spread. On January 14, the chief of WHO's Emerging Disease Unit acknowledged "it is possible there is limited human-to-human transmission . . . but it is very clear right now that we have no sustained human-to-human transmissions."

The WHO published a tweet that day:

Preliminary Investigations Conducted by the Chinese
Authorities Have Found No Clear Evidence of Human-to-
Human Transmission of the Novel #Coronavirus (2019-NCoV)
Identified in #Wuhan, #China.

This tweet was sent in spite of the testimonies from Taiwan and Dr. Ho that health care workers were getting the virus from patients, a blatant warning that human-to-human transmission was in fact occurring.

The same day the WHO was pooh-poohing the possibility of

human-to-human transmission, important CCP officials were gathering for an urgent teleconference. The Associated Press reported that, per internal CCP documents they had acquired, Ma Xiaowei, the head of China's National Commission of Health, informed the CCP leadership that they believed "the risk of transmission and spread [was] high" due to the upcoming Spring Festival travel season.

In response, according to the House Foreign Affairs Committee report, "The National Health Commission sent provincial health officials a 63-page instruction manual on how to respond to the outbreak, including requiring doctors and nurses to wear personal protective equipment. The instructions were marked 'internal' and 'not to be publicly disclosed.'"

All the while, the rest of the world was a sitting duck under the assumption there was no strong evidence of human-to-human spread and China was containing the virus. The congressional report continued:

> On January 17th the first new case since January 5th was announced, the day after the annual sessions of the Wuhan and Hubei provincial legislative and advisory bodies concluded. It should be noted that these political events began on January 6th, indicating announcements of new cases may have been suspended in order to not disrupt a major CCP political assembly.
>
> The next day, during this undisclosed public health response period, 40,000 families attended Lunar New Year–themed potluck banquets across the city of Wuhan.

President Xi Jinping finally warned the public of the coronavirus outbreak January 20 following the legislative meetings and holiday gatherings. This was six days after he was notified about the possibility of an epidemic, a timeline only admitted to in late February. However, by the time of the notice, more than 3,000 people had reportedly been infected during the week of public silence, according to documents obtained by The Associated Press and case approximations drawn from retrospective infection data.

By January 20, China and Western Pacific regional WHO offices were traveling to the area to begin their own investigation. It wasn't until then that the National Health Commission confirmed human-to-human transmission of the virus was occurring, despite warnings to the CCP a month prior.

It was clear that China's inflexible control of information and an unwillingness to send disparaging information up the chain of command shut down early warnings.

The report conceded there *was* indeed human-to-human transmission but cautioned more analysis was needed. The "more analysis needed" phrase seems to be a recurring theme throughout this pandemic, with many examples highlighted in this book, which begs the question: Is it better to get the initial, preliminary and unverified information out to the public earlier, risking retroactively correcting the communication, or is it better to delay information waiting for hard evidence confirming the issues? Was the warning of interhuman transmission delayed because intense scientific analysis was being performed, or was it a reprehensible effort to maintain favorable optics in front of watchful geopolitical foes?

A SHORT HISTORY OF CHINESE SCIENCE

Demonizing China is not going to help us get at the truth. It may help temporarily with the emotional turmoil people are facing during this time of crisis, but it does little to push us toward progress after the fact. Indeed, the heroic efforts of early Chinese whistleblowers and the Chinese people should inspire us all. Had they not been censored, their efforts would have had an even larger impact on alerting the world.

Without trying to explain away the CCP response to the virus, we can try to place it in historical context.

Until the late 1970s, China was largely cut off from the world, and with it the global flow of cutting-edge scientific knowledge. Chinese medical research and medical care were substandard and uneven at best. In significant parts of the country, especially in rural areas, people often went without vaccinations or regular access to medical professionals.

Once China began to open up to the world and undergo reform under the leadership of Deng Xiaoping, wealth streamed into the country. China had to make up for the mini–Dark Ages it had entered under Mao Zedong, in which intellectuals and researchers (and millions of others) suffered greatly from CCP oppression.

In the new, post-1978 era of Opening Up and Reform, China sought to recover its pride as an actively engaged player in world affairs, and to rival and eventually surpass the United States.

Science was absolutely crucial to this effort. As such, science and politics became dangerously entangled.

As the economy exploded, money flowed into research labs. Western scientists were courted and lavishly funded, while China sought to transform itself into a force to be reckoned with. The scientific turn in Opening Up and Reform–era China was not, however, purely political. The traditional Chinese love for education, which had been so painfully thwarted during the anti-intellectual Cultural Revolution, in which teachers were routinely humiliated and even violently attacked, doubtless played a role in that turn.

Yet even as money gushed into the endeavor of converting China into a global scientific research powerhouse during the 1990s and 2000s, the norms that underlie such research—namely, openness and transparency—proved difficult for the CCP, which depends upon concealment in order to cover up its ruthless treatment of dissenters and obfuscation to protect the fictions that it propounds about itself.

Today, the world wants the CCP to take responsibility for their obscuration of information and to let the truth come out. One study concluded that China might have been able to limit their own infections by up to 95 percent if the CCP had acted in late December, when heroic doctors were first raising the alarm. While we are grateful to the courageous whistleblowers, this is a cautionary tale of listening to people on the ground and lessening reliance on governmental reporting.

But the CCP, unfortunately, may not be able to handle the truth. While it shells out lavish funding and accolades to scientists, science itself—a clear, standardized, replicable inquiry into truth—represents standards that the party cannot allow to spread internally, lest its political system collapse. The dichotomy of an enigmatic government and the transparency of true academia will eternally collide, with political provocation always undermining scientific discovery.

A paper published in the *Proceedings of the National Academy of Sciences* found that by January 12, 2020, the daily risk of exporting a single case of COVID-19 to a country outside of China exceeded 95 percent and the likely first export occurred sometime in December 2019. Yet, the Chinese government didn't impose travel restrictions out of Wuhan to the rest of China until January 23, 2020. A fatal error.

Today's China is a beacon for scientists around the world in some limited senses, and a cautionary tale in others. *Western nations' key mistake is a profound ambivalence and lack of action in the face of growing warnings.* And the consequence of the unpursued ambivalence toward China with respect to the cover-up of SARS-CoV-2 has been untold suffering for the world.

By China's not sharing viral samples, the clear evidence of early human-to-human transmission, and subsequent underreporting of the spread of the virus, the world was dependent on China's misinformation. That reliance kept China from being isolated and discarded and because of such actions, the virus escaped, resulting in a global pandemic killing over 3 million people worldwide.

China's story is a great example of how dangerous it is when science is politicized.

FROM CHINA TO THE WORLD

On January 23, 2020, WHO Director-General Dr. Tedros Adhanom Ghebreyesus made a fateful decision. He decided not to declare a public health emergency of international concern (PHEIC), stating, "This is an emergency in China, but it has not yet become a global health emergency. At this time, there is *no* evidence of human-to-human transmission outside China."

The same day Dr. Tedros chose not to declare a public health emergency, the CCP implemented a citywide quarantine in Wuhan, halting all public transportation in and out of the city to other places in China. All this occurred while travel from China to other countries throughout the world did not cease. The virus was set loose across the globe. *Voice of America* estimates that 5 million people had fled Wuhan in the weeks preceding.

The WHO's message came despite confirmed cases outside of the PRC, cases among health care staff within the PRC, warnings from Taiwan and the University of Hong Kong, and knowledge that viruses do not respect geographical boundaries between people who are within China and those who are outside its borders.

Yet, censorship of media and whistleblowers, delayed presentation of information to the WHO, and obstruction disallowing the U.S. CDC to do an independent investigation kept the world in the dark about the human-to-human transmission occurring.

The same day the statement was released, the first case of COVID-19 in the United States was reported in a man who had just returned home from Wuhan.

How many times do we have to go through the same exhaustive routine? In an attempt to keep favorable optics, the Chinese kept secret information crucial for controlling and mitigating the growing outbreak, exactly what occurred nearly two decades earlier with the original SARS-CoV crisis.

The CCP later banned group travel abroad but permitted individuals to travel, as though the novel virus infected only large groups and not individuals. The announcement came 17 days after massive outbound traffic for the Spring Festival had begun.

In the ensuing days, various other countries across the globe, including France, Australia, and Canada, reported their first cases of COVID-19.

Eventually, the Chinese lockdown that followed included neighborhood groups, with grassroots-level enforcement of strict stay-at-home orders, even limiting how often people could leave their homes to purchase necessary provisions. Peter Hessler, a professor at the nearby Sichuan University, described in *The New Yorker* in early August 2020 that, "If a family were suspected of exposure to the virus, it wasn't unheard-of for their door to be sealed shut while tests and contact-tracing were being conducted."

One would think that the same central government that eventually demonstrated its ability to marshal resources and build makeshift hospitals in a week could have moved more quickly to stop the spread of the virus earlier, had they been less concerned with maintaining the appearance of being in total control of the situation.

THE UNDERCOUNT

To further add to the misperception that the virus was under control, the new case and death counts being reported from China were often suspected to be deliberate underestimates.

While China eventually imposed a strict lockdown to counter the rising infection rates, there has been considerable skepticism toward China's stated numbers, from both outside and within the country. While the world was experiencing drastically rising cases, it was becoming obvious that case and fatality rates being reported from China may have been inaccurate.

The precise number itself makes little difference in the grand scheme of things; the bigger picture regarding the counts is what mattered. Higher case numbers, faster doubling time, and more deaths would have informed the concern level in other countries, which then may have resulted in faster and stricter control measures.

In early April, the U.S. intelligence community concluded in a classified report issued to the White House that China had concealed the extent of the coronavirus outbreak, underreporting both total cases and deaths. The thrust of the report was that China's public reporting on cases and deaths was intentionally incomplete. Two of the officials said that the report concludes China's numbers were outright falsified.

In an off-the-record phone interview in June 2020 with a senior-level U.S. federal government medical professional, my source indicated that the United States had a counsel in Wuhan who reported people lined up in droves waiting to get through the doors of the hospital to be seen by health care workers in February. This coincides with whistleblower and other eyewitness accounts.

Further contributing to the conflict between government statements and tangible evidence, Bloomberg News reported thousands of urns were stacked outside funeral homes in Hubei province. While the world had their own skepticism, local public doubt in Beijing's reporting was also growing.

In late March, Radio Free Asia interviewed residents of Wuhan who said the CCP's official death toll of 2,500 was suspiciously low. The interview suggested the Hankou Funeral Home received a batch of 5,000 new urns in a single day, while seven other locally prominent funeral homes in Wuhan were reportedly returning the remains of approximately 500 people to their families each day.

Prior to mid-February, the only cases being reported by the CCP were those that were symptomatic and confirmed by laboratory tests. On February 13, NPR stated the reporting standards were expanded to include those unable to get a test or who had been tested with results still pending. Immediately following this policy change, the CCP reported an exasperating 14,840 new cases in one day.

Detailed in records released a month later was classified data showing by the end of February roughly 43,000 additional asymptomatic people in China had tested positive for the virus. However, they had not been included in the official reported case counts because, since they were asymptomatic, they were not being publicly disclosed initially.

It was not until the last day in March, after it became public knowledge that asymptomatic and presumptive cases were not being disclosed, that this policy was reversed. In April, Wuhan officials revised their estimated deaths up 50 percent.

As we have come to find out on our own, asymptomatic and presymptomatic spread of the virus is a major contributor to the transmission of SARS-CoV-2. Thus, omission of this information would have resulted in delayed and underperforming international preparedness and responses.

"The reality is that we could have been better off if China had been more forthcoming," Vice President Mike Pence said in an interview on CNN in early April 2020. "What appears evident now is that long before the world learned in December that China was dealing with this, and maybe as much as a month earlier than that, that the outbreak was real in China."

But, as Bloomberg reporters pointed out, "China isn't the only country with suspect public reporting. Western officials have pointed to Iran, Russia, Indonesia, and especially North Korea . . . as probable undercounts." Undercounts are not necessarily nefarious or intentional, rather testing ability and access to diagnostic capability can influence the ability to accurately count cases.

Conversely, in mid-April 2020, the former head of Britain's MI6 foreign intelligence service gave no allowance for the underreporting and said China intentionally "concealed crucial information about the novel coronavirus outbreak from the rest of the world and so should answer for its deceit," according to Reuters.

Some defenders of China say the Chinese waited to warn the public to fend off hysteria while behind the scenes they had been taking action. However, the whistleblower accounts suggest that may not have been the case, as alerting medical professionals and hospitals would have had tremendous results to lessen the amount of hospital-acquired infections. Notifying the public would have resulted in individual mitigation efforts to halt transmission among people as well.

CHINA'S PRIORITY: MAINTAINING GOOD OPTICS

Our global outbreak response system depends on the full participation and transparency of all participants. For authoritarian regimes, concealment is key to the maintenance of domestic power, and it's worth noting the intensification of Xi Jinping–era crackdowns on intellectual, religious, and personal freedoms that had been allowed in the Reform and Opening Up of China that began in 1978 under then-chairman Deng Xiaoping.

In China today, the rampant materialism and, more importantly, the focus on being world leaders in the field of science that were the hallmark goals of the Reform and Opening Up period are very much still intact. As the world's second largest economy, China devotes massive resources to scientific research and development, even going so far as to provide grounds for accusations of treason by prominent U.S. scientists, such as Harvard's Dr. Charles Lieber, and intellectual theft on an unimaginable scale. Today, the freedoms associated with the opening up era are eroding, as manifested by the political unrest in Hong Kong, outrage at the treatment of Uyghur Muslims, anger at pervasive corruption, and belligerent blame-mongering.

With respect to SARS-CoV-2, the CCP maintains that it saved the world from a virus that did not originate in Wuhan wet markets or in its labs, but the evidence indicates otherwise. It also suggests that the Chinese Communist Party acted to prevent word of the mystery illness from being shared. It took brave whistleblowers, leaked rumors, and the conscientiousness of small but mighty Taiwan and Singapore to alert the world to the seriousness of the outbreak. It almost didn't happen. Efforts were made to silence those sounding the alarm, as discovered by Lotus Ruan in a Citizen Lab publication. They reported that technology services began censoring keywords related to the outbreak, such as "unknown Wuhan pneumonia" and "Wuhan Seafood Market." This censorship campaign began on the same day the WHO was alerted of the online reports of the outbreak, December 31.

While omission of information itself is wrong, concealment is indefensible. The Chinese destroyed evidence, punished whistleblowers, and withheld the truth from the world and its own citizens on the eve of the biggest holiday travel season in the world. And yet Democrat leaders like Andrew Cuomo make sure to call COVID-19 the "European virus." CNN declared that the term "Chinese virus" was "inaccurate and is considered stigmatizing." We should always be careful to steer away from Sinophobia and to trumpet the accomplishments of the many brave Chinese people who fought to give us the truth during the pandemic—but the CCP bears enormous blame and the U.S. media should not let its biases blind it to this truth. Truly being pro-science means putting our political ideology to the side, being transparent, and following the facts where they lead.

CHAPTER 11

MISGUIDANCE FROM THE WORLD HEALTH ORGANIZATION

Men of science have made abundant mistakes of every kind; their knowledge has improved only because of their gradual abandonment of ancient errors, poor approximations, and premature conclusions.

—GEORGE SARTON

The labyrinthine, often bloated structure of large organizations tasked with holding nations in check makes it hard to place blame on them when they fail, for the same reason it makes it easy for the organizations to garner praise when they succeed.

There are so many layers to bureaucracy that it is easy to pick scapegoats (the proverbial "bad apples") and to blame the failure of an entire organization on one division or even one individual within it. Conversely, when such a corporation does something correct, the success of individuals or units within it is chalked up to the larger context in which their success occurred. Notoriously, though, information is unevenly distributed in huge organizations to the point that, if they had hands, we could rightly say of them that the left hand doesn't know what the right hand is doing. Indeed, some argue that huge institutions thrive precisely because they keep individuals hyper-focused so that obliviousness of the larger objective is rampant.

The World Health Organization (WHO), founded in 1948 by the United Nations, is nothing if not complex and bloated. As scholar Amy Staples notes in her book *The Birth of Development* on the post-WWII history of international development, even as early as 1949, the former USSR (itself no stranger to excessive bureaucracy) and the Republics of Ukraine and Byelorussia tried to opt out of membership on the grounds that the WHO was ineffective and that its "swollen administrative machinery" made it impossible to fund satisfactorily.

It is probably not a good sign when an organization has such structural problems that several of its members profess themselves ready to bail out the very next year after its formation.

Over its almost 75-year history, the WHO has had notable successes, perhaps most remarkably in the eradication of the highly fatal smallpox in 1980. Although the WHO cannot take sole credit for this accomplishment, we can say that it did not actively hinder the success of the joint effort by the USSR and the United States, launched in 1967 and completed ten years later, in eradicating the illness. While every hero story has a reprehensible undertone, it should be noted that at the same time that the USSR was collaborating with the United States to cure smallpox, they were also, as historian Erez Manela notes in *Diplomatic History*, designing a version of smallpox to use as a biological weapon. Wonderful as collaboration by scientific superpowers to fight the common enemy of disease is, it does not signify the end of political warfare.

As a product of the post-WWII enthusiasm for global organizations, the WHO was a child of its historical moment. That is as true now as it always has been; thus, it is not surprising that the WHO's current failures and successes reflect the intensifying struggle between the world's sole hegemon, the United States, and the rising superpower that is Communist China.

To be blunt, with respect to SARS-CoV-2, as we shall discuss in this chapter, the WHO—at least at the level of its leadership—seemingly failed to carry out its mission to monitor for global public health risks, prepare a coordinated response to the emerging situation, and provide information to promote human health and well-being. The WHO's inept bureaucracy and fawning relationship with China led it to make important blunders in the earliest days of the pandemic. Their closeness with China helped the authoritarian regime hoodwink the world as to the virus's true deadliness, and squandered valuable time. The WHO credulously believed China's misinformation about human-to-human transmission and opposed travel bans. The WHO is a prime example of what happens when a scientific organization is politicized completely.

Yet, any critic of the WHO is widely viewed as being anti-science and against public health.

If any other organization or employee had a perceived 100 percent failure rate on a project, they would be forced out of business or be fired. Still, there are many in academic communities who tout the organization as a beacon of unadulterated necessity and only profess praise for it in the name of science and global health. Also, never missing an opportunity to make themselves the center of attention, a large number of American celebrities fell all over themselves publicly praising the WHO, as did many mainstream media outlets. While applause for its historic work is warranted, not acknowledging areas of letdown undermines the credibility of the praise.

Central to the current criticism of the WHO is a series of missteps, full of lost opportunities and changing timelines, questioning the organization's commitment to its duty to protect. The disruption in the global economy and over 3 million lives lost also have people curious about political interference as the WHO's focus on appeasing their member state, China, seemed to guide some of its actions.

While science will always have a history full of blunders before reported success, the truth to be sought is whether political meddling resulted in actions contributing to the global devastation caused by COVID-19. If so, how many lives were lost from such blunders? A simple question with a complex answer, if there is to even be an answer.

In an attempt to explore and wholly understand what has occurred, it is fundamental to step back and understand the history of the WHO, its relationships with member states, and the timeline of their SARS-CoV-2 response.

In this chapter, I will consider the ways in which the WHO has been criticized throughout history and the course of the current pandemic for its seeming divergence from norms of the scientific community. Furthermore, we will discuss the devastation that may have been prevented had the organization acted independently of its member states.

Arguably, the WHO's botches derive from a problem that has come up over and over again in this book: the uneasy relationship between the needs of politics and the requirements of science. More specifically, the WHO, despite the high aims that inspired its founding back in 1948, has fallen hostage to political influence in the form of widespread cronyism and a bad habit of doing business with—and indeed, favoring—dictators and private industry interests. The title of a book that came out in 1997, *Le OMS: Bateau ivre de la santé publique* (*The WHO, the drunken sailor of public health*), edited by journalist Bertrand Deveaud and professor of economics Bertrand Lemennicier, perhaps sums up the esteem in which the WHO is held among those familiar with its inner workings.

THE HISTORY OF THE WHO

Of all histories of the post-WWII world, perhaps the one most likely to induce melancholia is that of the grandiose global organizations founded in the mid- to late 1940s. The United Nations (UN), and its offshoot the WHO were created to prevent war and disease from ever laying ruin to large portions of the world's peoples again. Everywhere, the emphasis shifted to the necessity of interdependence of the world and the need for shared attention to concerns that affected all members of the human family, or, as the famous photographic exhibition at the Museum of Modern Art that ran from January 24 to May 8, 1955 dubbed it, "The Family of Man."

Dr. George Brock Chisholm, a Canadian psychiatrist, served from 1946 onward as the executive secretary of the health committee that preceded the formation of the WHO, and was elected as its inaugural director-general in 1948. To his mind, the organization would bring doctors and scientists together from around the world to promote and defend health. Health, he defined as "a state of complete physical, mental and social well-being and not merely the absence of disease or infirmity."

Since "social well-being" inarguably is heavily dependent on the political state of a nation, the door was implicitly open for the politicization of the WHO's efforts from the start. Immediately, communist delegates began claiming Westerners were profit-driven in their quest for science, and Westerners made similarly pejorative claims about their non-liberal peers.

The original expectation was that the WHO would receive funds only from United Nations members. A few years ago, however, the organization set up what it calls a "private partnership" that allows financial support from private industries as well. As such, it has opened itself up to criticism of being swayed by its private connections as much as by its political sponsors.

GROWING DISTRUST STARTED WITH "BIRD FLU"

Cynicism about the WHO far precedes COVID-19, with the most notable criticism arising during the past avian flu pandemics.

During the 2009 bird flu outbreak, narratives arose calling attention to potential alliances among powerful actors, as well as less deceptive histories suggesting an element of public betrayal by the WHO. These stories were not wholly original, rather they were built upon a larger set of beliefs about trust and public health.

A joint investigation by the *British Medical Journal* (*BMJ*) and the Bureau of Investigative Journalism uncovered troubling questions about how the WHO managed conflicts of interest among scientists who advised its 2009 pandemic planning, and about the transparency of its advice to governments. The *BMJ* article reported that key scientists advising the World Health Organization during this time had done paid work for pharmaceutical companies manufacturing vaccines whose success hinged upon the WHO's declarations.

While the amalgamation of public health scientists and biomedical manufacturing is not foreign, transparency of such relationships is essential to oust disparagement. However, conflicts of interest between the WHO scientists and vaccine production companies were not disclosed. Further adding fuel to the incredulity, the WHO dismissed criticism of its handling of the A/H1N1 pandemic as mere anti-science conspiracy theories.

CANCELED. ANTI-SCIENCE. SOUND FAMILIAR?

Healthy skepticism in science is crucial, and should not be dismissed. By being unconvinced, one rejects complacency and lessens partiality in the quest for truth, modeling the real world as best as is possible.

The sequence of events during the avian flu pandemic only further contributed to the anti-vaccine movement and the overarching beliefs that these multinational organizations are in cahoots for profit at the expense of the general population. These beliefs—along with broader accounts of incidences undermining public trust—can have dangerous implications during a pandemic and onward.

The combination of popular skepticism about the efficacy of vaccines in general—combined with media coverage and erroneous celebrity stories—led people to doubt health authorities and, by extension, the WHO for its role in declaring H1N1 to be a pandemic. By declaring it as such, there was a strong push for vaccine manufacturing and stockpiling despite the virus's exceedingly low fatality rate, leaving people questioning whether a vaccine was necessary at all.

The lack of transparency by the WHO over the conflicts of interest, the documented change in the pandemic definition, and unanswered questions about the science behind certain therapeutic interventions all incited the emergence of such conspiracies.

Even people inside the WHO have publicly acknowledged internal corruption. Following the publication of a damning article in *The Lancet*, Dr. Tikki Pang, former director of Research Policy & Cooperation at the WHO, said his WHO colleagues were surprised by *The Lancet*'s study. However, Dr. Pang wholly acknowledged the criticism had merit:

> We know that our credibility is at stake. The lack of time and the shortage of information and of money can sometimes compromise the work of the WHO.

Following these events, the WHO's credibility has remained subject to scrutiny and its independence continues to be seriously questioned.

While the rank-and-file professionals working at the WHO may be doing their best, their efforts are being dwarfed by problems with the organization's leadership. Good intentions and dutiful work by many are not enough for a multibillion-dollar organization tasked with ensuring the public health and safety of the globe.

FORMING ALLIANCES WITH CHINA

The World Health Organization was intended to pool the world's resources with respect to medical science and promote human unity.

Unfortunately, the collapse of the WHO as a reliable guarantor of global health stems in part from being divided along political lines from the outset. This was particularly apparent in its selection of leadership. Indeed, as a 2016 article from the *American Journal of Public Health* rightly notes, "the WHO's leadership challenges can be traced to its first decades of existence."

Nowhere are the leadership challenges of the WHO more pressing than with respect to the current director-general, Tedros Adhanom Ghebreyesus, who was the favorite candidate of the Obama administration to lead the organization. Tedros's appointment decisions as director have made headlines throughout his tenure. For example, in 2017, he appointed Zimbabwe's Robert Mugabe as a WHO goodwill ambassador. As the BBC reported, Human Rights Watch said that it was an embarrassment to give the ambassador role to Mr. Mugabe, because his "utter mismanagement of the economy has devastated health services." After much criticism, Tedros gave up his plan to appoint Mugabe, but his praise of the Zimbabwean spoke volumes about his willingness to flatter and craft alliances with dictators.

Early on in his tenure, it became clear that Tedros had forged an alliance of sorts with China. The day after he was elected, Tedros reaffirmed his adherence to the "One China" doctrine by not inviting Taiwan for formal participation in the WHO, as China still claims it to be their territory. Because the WHO is, as one high-ranking U.S. intelligence expert speaking off the record put it, "in China's pocket," it is especially prone to putting out stories that support such narratives, whether or not they are accurate.

This brings to light one of the biggest weaknesses of the WHO, which is that it relies on truthful information from member countries.

Still reeling from the panic and fallout from the 2003 SARS pandemic as reports of a mystery illness in China began circulating in late 2019, Taiwan and Hong Kong could not help but remember that China had a long history of covering up epidemics. The health authorities in Taiwan and Hong Kong had a broad and deep understanding of the political complexities involving an outbreak, and of the relationship between the WHO and China, from prior experience.

Taiwan disregarded narratives from Chinese officials and the WHO that came out in early 2020. Instead, Taiwanese officials insisted that their population wear masks immediately. Taiwan also ignored the WHO's position that travel bans were dangerous and could incite xenophobia, as they closed their borders. For its part, Hong Kong began aggressively screening and isolating travelers as well. By discounting the information from the WHO, these countries immediately decreased the influx of virus while also mitigating the already infected.

Taiwan, forbidden from WHO membership, began sounding the alarm to the world. Imagine if the WHO had heeded their warnings rather than placating the CCP. Thankfully for them, Singapore, Taiwan, and Hong Kong paid no attention to the information being relayed by the WHO. As such, Taiwan currently has one of the lowest mortality burdens in the world.

A WHO report did not mention delays in information sharing or question the material being distributed by the CCP. It did say that "China's bold approach to contain the rapid spread of this new respiratory pathogen has changed the course of a rapidly escalating and deadly epidemic." The message to the world was that the WHO was largely satisfied with the information China was giving them and that the disease was essentially under control.

The precise moment at which members of the CCP and the WHO were provided evidence of human-to-human transmission is unknown, but it is safe to assume that it was far earlier than when they alerted everyone else. This wait had monumental repercussions. If the virus was dangerous enough to merit a ban on travel from Wuhan to destinations within China, why was it decided that it was acceptable to expose the world beyond the borders of China?

Unfortunately, the rest of the world was reliant on the misinformation and preparations were delayed.

Indeed, three critical weeks during the largest global migration holiday season passed before the WHO acknowledged an outbreak was occurring and there was human-to-human transmission, and then only after China was forced to disclose it by leaked information.

CONCEALING HUMAN-TO-HUMAN TRANSMISSION

Perhaps the first, and most pronounced, blunder since the emergence of the novel coronavirus was the WHO not alerting the world to reports suggesting SARS-CoV-2 was capable of being transmitted among humans.

Officials in Taiwan claim to have reported signs of human-to-human transmission to the International Health Regulations, a WHO information exchange network between 196 countries, on December 31, 2019, following hearsay from doctors that an outbreak was occurring. However, this alert was not shared with other countries, according to an interview with a Taiwan official by the *Financial Times*.

As a multilateral organization that lacks enforcement authority over its member states, the WHO cannot directly access countries' health information and therefore relies on them to provide it. However, the independence of the WHO may rightly be put into question when they openly disseminate information without query, despite evidence indicating that such information is false.

The WHO should have demanded early access to Wuhan, its hospitals, and whistleblower physicians to get a factual account of what was occurring. When independent access to Wuhan was denied as cases were rising, instead of regurgitating what China was claiming without contest, the WHO could have, at the very least, alerted the world that a situation was unfolding and highlighted the fact that they had not been allowed autonomous review.

It all could have happened the first week of January.

But it did not.

Despite the warnings in late December and early into January, in mid-January the WHO posted a tweet on its Twitter account downplaying the transmissibility of the outbreak:

> Preliminary investigations conducted by the Chinese authorities have found no clear evidence of human-to-human transmission of the novel #coronavirus (2019-nCoV) identified in #Wuhan, #China.

It wasn't until January 28, 2020, that Director-General Tedros traveled to Beijing as part of a WHO mission to assess the situation. At this time, he once again praised the handling of the outbreak by the Chinese Communist Party, citing the "transparency they have demonstrated, including sharing data and genetic sequence of the virus."

We were all fed the proverbial garbage that China had been forthcoming with information and genetic sequencing. Nowhere in his comments did Director-General Tedros note that much of the information was provided only after it was leaked online, that virus samples were not being provided, and that the CCP was not allowing independent investigations.

The WHO's global health emergency was finally declared on January 30, when there were already 115 confirmed cases outside of China.

On January 31, 2020, the White House gave an update on the situation saying that Chinese health officials had reported approximately 10,000 confirmed cases of the novel coronavirus in China, more than the total number of cases of severe acute respiratory syndrome (SARS) during its 2003 outbreak.

OPPOSING TRAVEL BANS

As infections were being reported outside of China, and with limited information coming from the WHO, on February 2, 2020,

President Trump enforced a limited travel ban on people who were coming from China into the United States, while exempting U.S. citizens and their families. At this time it was thought there were only a few cases in the United States, all with recent travel from China. Little did we know then that the virus had likely been here for weeks.

The ban by the United States slowed the spread of the virus by limiting the influx of new cases; however, it was implemented too late. Notably, the ban was made in the face of considerable political resistance by those who, at least initially, deemed it premature, xenophobic, racist, and ineffectual, and it was criticized by the WHO.

Two days after the ban was announced, Tedros stated measures that "unnecessarily interfere with international travel and trade" were not needed, despite evidence that the virus was spreading across multiple continents.

In a press briefing several days after the travel ban had been initiated, China's foreign ministry spokeswoman, Hua Chunying, even cited the WHO's advice, which discouraged countries from imposing travel restrictions on China, based on the organization's recognition of China's significant efforts to combat the virus. Hua further criticized the United States of "causing and spreading panic."

How could these statements not open up the discussion of political motivation of the WHO? The assertion was in direct response to the U.S. travel ban, yet ignored the fact that many other countries were not only doing the same thing, but were much more restrictive. Ultimately, those with harsher restraints had lower viral loads during the initial wave of the pandemic.

While a total travel ban might have made a much larger dent in controlling the spread to the United States, modeling and expert opinion suggests that even the partial travel ban delayed the spread, giving time to prepare for the rise of contagion. Ultimately, though, an *earlier* ban would have stopped the virus from escaping China. Yet, the WHO continued to echo misinformation that further fumbled the response efforts during that short window of opportunity to contain the virus.

DISCOURAGING MASK USE

The travel ban bought some time to gather personal protective equipment (PPE) for health care workers and maximize available hospital beds. Concurrently, the CDC and WHO were recommending *against* the general public wearing face masks, partly predicated on the supposed low disease prevalence of the virus as reported by China.

A reasonable concern regarding public usage of masks was the limited supply of surgical masks and N95 respirators for health care professionals and infected patients. At this time, experts didn't know how easily the virus spread between people without symptoms or how long infectious particles could linger in the air, so the recommendation against generalized use of masks in asymptomatic people seemed appropriate.

Up until that moment, the science behind generalized mask-wearing was actually not supportive of it. In fact, many research trials, including randomized-controlled ones, studying the use of cloth masks concluded they should *not* be used because of the false sense of security of wearing them. Some smaller studies looking at influenzas and coronaviruses from a population level have shown a decrease in viral transmission, not elimination, through generalized wearing of face masks. But again, most studies advocating against, or even for, cloth masks have been done to evaluate influenza viruses, and the novel coronavirus has proven to be quite different from influenza.

So, preceding COVID-19, the science was mixed but leaned more away from widespread public mask-wearing as a means to slow transmission.

Thus, for months the World Health Organization declined to

recommend mask-wearing, partly out of supply concerns and worry people wouldn't wear masks properly, giving them a false sense of security, none of which has been documented to have played out in Hong Kong or other mask-wearing places.

Because the informed risk of transmission was low initially, as reported by the CCP, the WHO continued to describe the transmission of SARS-CoV-2 from asymptomatic people as "rare." Therefore, if someone was sick, it made sense to have them isolate while the medical care personnel could equip themselves with adequate PPE to care for them.

However, a key component to this virus that the WHO delayed acknowledging is an alternate route of transmission. The agency's pandemic response team came under fire months later, according to STAT News, "when more than 200 scientists accused the WHO in an open letter of resisting evidence that virus-laced aerosols— emitted by people infected with Covid-19—[were] fueling spread of the disease," rather than it being spread solely by respiratory droplets.

The WHO has long maintained that SARS-CoV-2 is spread via larger respiratory droplets, like other coronaviruses and influenza, while it repeatedly dismissed the possibility of more ubiquitous airborne aerosol transmission. Respiratory droplets are heavy and drop to the floor faster, are easier to contain, and are often found when someone sneezes, coughs, or spits; whereas aerosol particles are exuded merely by breathing and speaking, lingering in the air much longer, making them highly more communicable.

The delayed recognition of airborne transmission and the deficiency of clear recommendations on control measures against an airborne virus had significant consequences. People may have mistakenly believed they were fully protected by adhering to the current recommendations when, in fact, additional airborne interventions were, and are, needed.

The rapid changing of recommendations, while not foreign to

scientific discovery, fuels distrust among those who are basing their lifestyles on such suggestions.

By early April, when U.S. physicians and researchers had a couple of months' worth of experience with SARS-CoV-2, U.S. public health leaders separated from the WHO and encouraged the general public to wear face masks. This marked an acknowledgment of the high propensity of transmission from asymptomatic and presymptomatic individuals and the potential for the virus to aerosolize.

Recommendations will always change as evidence becomes available, especially for a new virus with limited data. However, when a grassroots organization and/or individual brings a discovery to the public's attention rather than the international authorities, this adds to the overall discord.

It wasn't until June when the WHO endorsed the generalized wearing of masks, only after overwhelming research-based evidence of aerosol transmission emerged and the virus was already spreading out of control throughout the world.

Their belatedness cost lives. However, by that time, few were listening to them anymore as their partisan support for China was evident.

THE WHO'S FUTURE

Less than four months after the novel coronavirus began spreading across the globe, President Trump announced that he would "terminate the relationship" with the World Health Organization if they did not "commit to major substantive improvements." During the announcement he accused the organization of grossly mismanaging the COVID-19 outbreak in its early stages, and inferred its allegiance to China by calling the organization "China-centric."

The United States is the top contributor to the organization, providing nearly $900 million for a two-year budget cycle, accounting for roughly 20 percent of the total contributions. With a budget of $4.8 billion for a two-year cycle, the United States plays a critical role in ensuring adequate support.

It was not immediately clear whether the intention was to solely withhold funding or if termination of the United States' membership would be sought. It is important to note that while the president has some authority to withhold membership status and dues, if Congress allocates international aid via a mandate the president lacks the ability to deny such funding.

The largest allocation ($863 million) of the upcoming 2020/2021 WHO funding goes toward polio vaccination efforts across the globe. A disease once greatly feared for its high rates of permanent paralysis and death, polio was eradicated in the western hemisphere in 1994. Today, the virus causing this illness is still circulating in regions across the world, including such countries as Pakistan and Nigeria. It is imperative to emphasize that many nations, especially poor ones, depend on the WHO for much of their health care, vaccination programs, and medical supplies. As we have seen with COVID-19, we are united in public health, as a virus does not respect geographic boundaries. If polio is not controlled in the areas where it remains endemic, and less of the global population receive the vaccine, we may have a resurgence of this devastating illness, among others.

While we can firmly acknowledge the need for the WHO, we can't be naïve about the challenges of keeping any would-be apolitical institution afloat in a world largely dominated by politics. Our leaders must also concede the WHO's response to this pandemic disappointed the world—as well as its own mission. It did not protect global health—rather, it contributed to imperiling it.

By the end of 2020, the United States was intentionally behind in its member dues and as 2021 began, it became evident that the defunding move would not carry forward. President-Elect Joe Biden vowed to continue the WHO funding once in office while also declaring he would ensure the CDC was stationed in other parts of the world. That is, assuming they allow us to be there.

But such a statement is hollow. The solution of simply providing more financial support and not condemning the WHO's inability to indict China's concealment actions is merely a form of political posturing.

All science, including public health science, is messy. So a level of humbleness must be present in the search for progress and improvement. There also must be a sense of pragmatism surrounding the corruption and shortcomings that consume an organization that is deeply flawed, but remains essential.

Looking ahead, repairing, not eliminating, the broken fundamentals of the WHO is critical, because developing countries, in particular, need a high-functioning global health provider. Without the U.S. contributions, the world would suffer. However, the world will also suffer if the WHO is not held accountable for its actions and is biting the so-called hand that feeds it.

We might turn to history, study in particular the success of the Smallpox Elimination Project, remembering that its success happened at the height of the Cold War, and that it depended on collaboration between rival superpowers.

This is not the place to address the million-dollar question of just how the WHO might be reimagined, but perhaps we might remember that the mechanisms for determining the leadership of organizations and their funding often explain much about their subsequent conduct. The "democracy deficit" that plagues big institutional organizations cannot be paid for in the loss of human life, as it has with respect to the WHO under Tedros.

If the WHO had been more accountable, independent, and mission-driven, we could have conceivably avoided a disastrous situation. Such an organization would not have praised China for its handling of the virus, even suggesting low viral transmission without performing its own investigation. A politically neutral organization certainly would not have remained silent when China imposed travel bans within its own borders while criticizing other countries for executing such bans against China.

In the same vein, an apolitical WHO should not have waited until mid-March before finally declaring a pandemic. By that point, 114 countries had already reported cases, and more than 4,000 confirmed deaths had occurred.

As China continues to grow its global economic stronghold, more and more countries are becoming wary of criticizing Beijing in fear of retaliation. The western hemisphere has taken to treating China with kid gloves to maintain relationships.

While China's concealment may have been the culprit, the WHO acted as an accomplice. Distrust of China already existed, but we trusted the WHO to protect the world by providing accurate information. We were blindsided.

However, should we have been? The alliance between the WHO and China was obvious, and it continues to play out today. All we must do to keep tabs on the allegiance is to observe the WHO's unrelenting treatment of Taiwan.

The loyalty can be perfectly summarized in the story of Yvonne Tong, a Hong Kong–based producer of *The Pulse*, an English-language news program. Her special interests are, as her personal website notes, in "human rights, inequality, law and order, as well as Hong Kong–China politics." She is known for her documentary work on Chinese ethnic minorities, such as the Uyghurs.

Back in April 2020, this young woman secured an interview with Bruce Aylward, the assistant director-general of the WHO. The BBC gave the following account of what happened when she asked a question about Taiwan:

> In the segment, Ms. Tong asks if the WHO would reconsider letting Taiwan join the organization. She is met with a long silence from Mr. Aylward, who then says he cannot hear her and asks to move on to another question. Ms. Tong presses him again, saying she would like to talk about Taiwan. At this

point, Mr. Aylward appears to hang up on her. When the journalist calls Mr. Aylward again, she asks if he could comment on Taiwan's response to the coronavirus.

Mr. Aylward then replies: "Well, we've already talked about China."

If the WHO is devoted to the health of all people in the world and is expected to be the pillar of science, it needs to be willing to work with everyone, without censorship—including those who go against the CCP red line. Pretending not to hear and hanging up won't work on tough questions about how to accommodate political differences in the service of the larger goal of global health. Neither will not listening work when it comes to criticism of the leadership and overall structure of the WHO—which, if the response to SARS-CoV-2 is any measure, is badly in need of reform, lest it do more harm to the people of the world.

Epidemiologists at Imperial College London estimated there were about 4,000 symptomatic cases in Wuhan by January 18, 2020. Other researchers published in *The Lancet* projected there were more than 75,000 cases in the locality by January 25, with thousands of infected cases exported on international flights during the first half of January 2020.

Had the WHO listened to Taiwan's warnings on December 31, 2019, and restricted travel from China then, over 5 million people would not have left Wuhan during the Chinese New Year celebrations. This single action might have saved hundreds of thousands of lives.

Even now, no strong measures have been made to ensure such blind support of the CCP won't harm the world again. The WHO must be held to task; the question is, who will do it? Decades of treating the CCP with kid gloves by the West and now present-day politics indicate neither will be held accountable for the deaths they caused.

CHAPTER 12

UPON AMERICAN SOIL

What Happened?

There was no stopping the virus from landing on American soil during the largest global migration of the Chinese New Year. However, were we to try to assess the response to SARS-CoV-2 once it arrived solely by mainstream media reports, we might come away with the sense that we are surrounded by villains on the right and on the left.

Panic, though, predictably hinges on partisan politics and more specifically, on which politician and party are to blame for the pandemic and for everything else, to boot. Complacency and poor preparation by preceding administrations meant we were left on the back foot when the virus arrived on our shores.

Truly, though, the story of the collective response to SARS-CoV-2 on American soil begins long before the first infected person flew into U.S. airspace from China.

Adequate preparedness for a pandemic, if there is such a thing, requires a preexisting infrastructure, a process that can take years to accomplish. Thus, the story of the American response to COVID-19 is best told over an extended period of time.

PANDEMIC PREPAREDNESS AND THE STOCKPILE

Back in 1999, the U.S. had established a Strategic National Stockpile (then known as the National Pharmaceutical Stockpile) of medical supplies to be used during emergencies.

The fundamental role of the stockpile is to support state and local officials during public health crises severe enough to deplete existing medical supplies. Essentially, the stockpile is supposed to function as a stopgap during disasters while production to replenish reinforcements can be ramped up.

It was in 2005 that the wheels were set in motion for what was to be a new era of pandemic preparedness. As ABC News reported, this was the year in which "the nation's most comprehensive pandemic plan—a playbook that included diagrams for a global early warning system, funding to develop new, rapid vaccine technology, and a robust national stockpile of critical supplies, such as face masks and ventilators—was created."

John Barry's *The Great Influenza: The Story of the Deadliest Pandemic in History* came out the preceding year, and President George W. Bush received a copy. Barry's book surveys the origins, consequences, and key figures in the 1918 flu pandemic, painting a harrowing portrait of human suffering and the human errors that made it worse.

The book was a wake-up call for POTUS, as President Bush took the content to heart. The message struck him so intensely that he immediately contacted homeland security advisor Fran Townsend and insisted that the country set a course for pandemic preparedness. At the time, Townsend said, her response was as follows: "My reaction was—I'm buried. I'm dealing with counterterrorism. Hurricane season. Wildfires. I'm like, 'What?' He said to me, 'It may not happen on our watch, but the nation needs the plan.' "

President Bush's response to Barry's book was surely conditioned by his then-recent memories of September 11, 2001, and of the anthrax attacks that shortly thereafter followed. Reading John Barry's book reminded him that the threat posed by infectious disease could arise from nature as well as from the intentional use of biological weapons. As such, he moved quickly to act, befitting his duties as a wartime president in the post-9/11 years.

Shortly thereafter, President Bush announced the National Strategy for Pandemic Influenza, which provided a high-level approach for the federal and local governments to take in order to prepare for and respond to a pandemic.

Essential and relatively affordable patient care supplies and medications meant for basic life support (face masks, intravenous fluids, oxygen, and antibiotics) were purchased first. More expensive, technologically advanced life support equipment (such as mechanical ventilators) was purchased later when additional funds became available.

In an interview given in 2020, Charles Johnson, president of International Safety Equipment Association, said by the time the 2009 flu crisis hit, the stockpile was stocked with about 100 million face masks. In an effort to protect frontline workers, according to a Centers for Disease Control report published following the 2009 pandemic, the Obama administration distributed 39 million of the N95 masks during the first wave of infections, followed by nearly 60 million more for the second wave.

However, when the crisis ended and nearly 100 million masks had been removed, the Obama administration decided not to wholly replenish what was taken out of the stockpile. Instead, they turned their focus on other measures, allotting $600 million to go toward items such as antiviral medications and flu vaccines.

While anti-flu drugs and vaccines play an important role in influenza epidemics, they are hardly relied upon as primary means of preparedness for other viral outbreaks. The reason being, the effectiveness of antiviral treatments and vaccines vary for each influenza season, not to mention, they are not effective for preventing and treating other respiratory viruses, such as the novel coronavirus.

Masks, on the other hand, will always be in demand and should have been restocked immediately.

Because the Strategic National Stockpile serves many purposes, it was not designed specifically with the idea of constant preparedness for infectious disease pandemics. Over time, threats to the U.S. national security expand and diversify continuously. And so, as the U.S. drifted toward 2020, the urgency of President Bush in 2005 had been forgotten through shifts in power and changing priorities. While Obama built upon the existing pandemic response unit, the additions were largely dismantled by the Trump administration. What was considered a national threat of maximum urgency one year became less substantial the following year, and budget decisions were made based on available information regarding the most prevalent threats.

As 2020 began and the COVID-19 pandemic was underway, the stockpile reportedly consisted of only 12 million N95 respirators and 30 million surgical masks—a supply considered to be less than 2 percent of what was estimated to be needed for a large-scale outbreak.

The time to replace the supply had expired, with neither the Obama nor Trump administrations replenishing it sufficiently. This neglect led to the frenzied situation where the country scrambled to obtain hundreds of millions of new masks in the midst of a pandemic.

CONTAINMENT

While preparedness is imperative for any crisis, containment is the first and foremost goal once a crisis begins. On January 19, 2020, the WHO Western Pacific Regional Office (WHO/WPRO) tweeted that, "according to the latest information received and WHO analysis, there was evidence of *limited* human-to-human transmission" (emphasis mine).

The following day, the WHO tweeted about information newly reported suggesting that there could be *sustained* human-to-human transmission.

Although those two messages may seem similar and redundant to many, there was a one-word change that made all the difference to people paying attention: *sustained*.

The single word change—from *limited* to *sustained*—had very important implications. It is much more challenging to control an outbreak with *sustained* human-to-human transmission than one with *limited* transmission.

The WHO defines *sustained* human-to-human transmission as easily transmitted from one person to the next. That's in contrast to *limited* human-to-human transmission, in which a virus dies out after infecting a person or a few people among clusters of people who are in close contact with each other, as in a domestic or a workplace setting.

Having had this warning from the WHO, the federal government began efforts to delay the introduction of the pathogen into the United States and contain it once it arrived. CDC officials announced enhanced symptom screening for travelers from Wuhan at three international airports, in Los Angeles, San Francisco, and New York, on January 17, several days before the WHO indicated sustained transmission was occurring. The screening of travelers was expanded to 20 U.S. airports within a week of the declaration of sustained transmission.

The transmissibility of a virus hangs on what is called its "basic reproduction number (R0)." This is a metric used to describe the contagiousness of infectious pathogens, such as viruses and bacteria. The R0 "R naught" is affected by numerous factors (biological, socio-behavioral, and environmental) that influence transmission and can even be influenced by human behaviors, highlighting how fluid and unpredictable science can be.

Built on the initial numbers reported from China, coupled with information about the demographics of the population in

Wuhan, the R0 was estimated as 1.5 to 2, meaning that every one person infected was expected to infect up to two other people. Seasonal flu has an R0 of approximately 1.3, meaning that even given documented sustained human-to-human transmission, harsh measures were probably not thought to be warranted as the novel virus's initial R0 predictions were not considered to be much higher than those for the flu. Of course, our calculation of the R0 was wholly dependent upon China being forthcoming with the amount of cases and we now know that the CCP was being anything but that.

The preceding SARS and MERS viruses had a respective R0 of 2 to 3, and less than 1. While not a coronavirus, the R0 for the earlier 2009 influenza virus was found to be 1.5.

Yet, as new cases of the novel coronavirus started to be reported throughout the eastern hemisphere in January 2020, it quickly became clear that the transmissibility of SARS-CoV-2 was much greater than was originally relayed by Chinese officials, with the CDC estimating the R0 ranging as high as 8.9.

The result of the misrepresentation of transmissibility was that countries such as Italy and other areas of Europe were knocked on their tails early on. With an estimated R0 lower than the original SARS and with the WHO praising China for their "transparency and containment" efforts, why would other countries expect anything other than containment of this, seemingly less contagious, coronavirus?

The world was preparing for a flu pandemic or regional SARS-like epidemic based on defective information, when they should have been preparing for something much more ominous. As the growing crisis gained more media attention, trepidation also began to grow. And when unease sets in, people tend not to stay in place unless they are forced to do so. Rather, they try to get out of the affected areas.

The New York Times reported that about 430,000 people flew on direct flights from China to the United States during January 2020.

Thousands of passengers came directly from the city of Wuhan. However, the report did not consider travelers who may have come into the U.S. on a connecting flight, thereby underrepresenting the number of people traveling from China to the United States during that crucial time.

By the third week of January, quite predictably, the United States and South Korea each reported their first cases of the novel coronavirus, both from people who recently traveled home from Wuhan, China.

A little over a week later, the first human-to-human transmission in the U.S. was recorded. The husband of a woman who had traveled home from Wuhan developed a fever, prompting testing. The virus had effectively made its way to establishing itself upon American soil.

THE TRAVEL BAN

As soon as it became clear that the R0 was being badly underestimated, the Trump administration made the decision to impose a travel ban on January 31, 2020.

Domestically, the travel ban prompted an immediate, highly partisan outcry. Former Vice President Joe Biden and House Speaker Nancy Pelosi were outspoken, with Biden tweeting in early March, "walls will not stop the coronavirus" and "banning travel from Europe—or any part of the world won't stop it." While Biden retroactively says he supported the travel ban restrictions imposed by Trump, after medical experts admitted that travel bans likely contributed to slowing the spread, the tweet raised questions as to the validity of the ban, polarizing Americans. Nancy Pelosi even walked through San Francisco's Chinatown in a publicity stunt saying, "But we do want to say to people, come to Chinatown, here we are. We're again careful, safe, and come join us."

By that time, though, 59 airline companies had suspended or limited flights to mainland China, and several additional countries—including Russia, Australia, and Italy—imposed travel restrictions from China, as the United States had done, also discouraging travel.

Making the decision to impose a travel ban is not an easy one. A complete shutdown of incoming flights to the United States would seemingly have had a more profound delay in the virus spread but would also have an economic implication that may have caused even more harm. Though when flights are shut down administratively, people eventually find a way around the ban through broken itineraries and make their way without the necessary screening and quarantines.

The initial travel bans undoubtedly slowed the early onslaught of cases.

Yet from a scientific perspective, the controversial bans may have been declared too late and may not have been harsh enough during the busiest international travel time of the year. By that time, the science has shown, the cases in the Northeast were primarily from a European strain of COVID-19.

Nearly 2 million travelers entered the United States from Europe in February as that continent became the new epicenter of the pandemic.

A retrospective study led by researchers at Northeastern University in Boston concluded that New York likely had more than 10,000 undetected cases by March 1. Infections reached critical mass in New York and other cities long before the mid-March Europe travel ban was instituted.

Unsurprisingly, immediately following the announcement of the Europe travel ban, a mass exodus of people (mostly those returning home) occurred from Europe to the United States.

The number of passengers arriving from the involved countries rose 46 percent on the day following the travel ban proclamation as people clambered to get home before the restrictions went into place, according to data from Customs and Border Protection and reported by *The Washington Post*.

A friend of mine involved in the mad dash to return to the U.S. from a European spring break vacation recounted the airport scene as "wholly chaotic." Airport employees were ushering passengers in herd-like fashion to their flights and offering alternate re-routes to get people home. Questions about symptoms were asked but there were no temperature checks and no formalized screening process, just pandemonium.

"We closed the front door with the China travel ban, but we left the back door wide open," New York governor Andrew M. Cuomo said during one of his now-famous daily press conferences. His statement inferred delaying the institution of a complete travel ban led to the growing enormity of the situation.

Like him or not, this was true.

On March 11, the World Health Organization finally declared the coronavirus a global pandemic as it was now occurring world-wide, crossing international boundaries and affecting a large number of people.

Officials turned a blind eye to what was going on in late winter, and even urged people to gather and socialize together. Indeed, City & State reported, "in February, de Blasio attempted to quash growing anti-Asian sentiments stemming from the disease's Chinese origins, by encouraging people to partake in Lunar New Year celebrations and dine in the city's Chinese neighborhoods." The goal was noble, I suppose, but diseases respect nobility as little as they care about nationality. People went out to bars and restaurants and mingled closely together. And with them went the virus.

The growing calamity also exposed a serious dysfunction playing out behind the scenes at a time when New Yorkers badly needed to have confidence in their local authority. That confidence was eroded daily by internal leaks and reported intra-agency infighting. The future of this city was—and still is, as of this writing—hanging in the balance. As City Council Speaker Corey Johnson said at an oversight hearing on City Hall's response to the COVID-19 outbreak, "New Yorkers deserve better."

In the response in New York, we can see the effect of bureaucratic mismanagement, lack of preparation causing shortages, and blunders that led to catastrophic consequences in nursing homes. All of this was followed by cover-ups on high, as Governor Cuomo tried to shift the conversation from his failed policies while still claiming that "New York follows the science."

A SHORTAGE OF HOSPITALS

Overnight, New York City and surrounding areas experienced sharp surges in the demand for medical services, which overwhelmed localities.

The proportion of symptomatic people that needed hospital admission was proving to be significantly higher for COVID-19 than for seasonal flu and even the 2009 influenza pandemic. Further, the risk of admission to the intensive care unit was discovered to be "five to six times higher in patients infected with SARS-CoV-2 than in" the H1N1 pandemic, according to a *Lancet* article published in July, which is why there was a growing concern for a critical need of ICU beds and ventilators. This all was occurring during the midst of flu season, when hospital capacity is already stretched thin.

Our medical system is well-equipped to deal with the routine challenges presented by infectious diseases around us. But anyone who studies hospitals—and indeed, the U.S. health care system more generally—knows what the problems are regarding hospitalization. Unfortunately, COVID-19 exposed areas of vulnerability within our system, including the drastic decrease in available hospital beds over the last two decades.

A series of legislative actions, including the Affordable Care Act, incentivized merging of health systems. This resulted in hospital unifications, combining wealth and authority and forcing closure of the smaller, less profitable hospitals.

This is not the place for a full-blown account of *that* issue. We can note, however, that following the expansion of Medicaid, New York was forced to close many hospitals, which left them vulnerable when it came time for the massive stress test of the pandemic.

The inception of the fallout of hospital services in New York began even earlier, in 2005, after Governor George Pataki created the Berger Commission. The group was formed after a state commission determined New York had an excess of inpatient hospital beds, which was contributing to excessive medical care expenditures. Following review, the Berger Commission agreed that there was a surplus of inpatient beds in New York State and recommended closure of nine hospitals, with downsizing or mergers of an additional 48 hospitals. In all, inpatient capacity was reduced by 7 percent, resulting in the loss of 4,000 beds.

Enter the Affordable Care Act and its accompanying Medicaid expansion. Governor Cuomo was a devoted supporter of the expansion, which increased Medicaid coverage for New York in 2014 with one in three residents being covered by the government program. While some of the measures were proven to be beneficial, it was found to cost more than expected. The expense of such comprehensive coverage left Cuomo working against a $6 billion deficit tied directly to the expansion. As a result, several smaller safety-net hospitals that primarily serve low-income populations closed or were forced to reduce services and inpatient beds.

In all, since 2003, 41 hospitals have closed in New York State, including 18 in New York City alone. Two decades ago there were 73,931 licensed hospital beds in New York State when there were 18.3 million people living there. By 2020, there were only 53,470 beds for a population that has grown to 19.4 million.

In November 2016, policy experts issued warnings of marginalizing care for the underserved that fell on deaf ears after New York's health system cut thousands of hospital beds in search of cost savings and efficiencies.

As COVID-19 hit New York City, Cuomo announced New York State had about half the amount of beds that was projected to be needed to adequately care for residents with COVID-19.

As *The Wall Street Journal* explained, "Only after the disease had gripped the city's low-income neighborhoods in early March did Gov. Cuomo and Mayor de Blasio mobilize public and private hospitals to create more beds and intensive-care units. The hasty expansion that ensued, led by New York government leaders and hospital administrators, produced mistakes that helped worsen the crisis, health-care workers say."

The Wall Street Journal also reported talking to "nearly 90 frontline physicians, nurses, hospital administrators and public health officials, and also reviewed emails and legal documents to analyze what went wrong." They reported, "Among the missteps identified, they uncovered insufficient isolation protocols which led to the mixing of infected patients with the uninfected, facilitating the spread of the virus. General hospital floors and outpatient areas were being outfitted to function as ICU space and various ventilation devices were retrofitted to increase supply of ventilators." The *Journal* also reported "inadequate staff availability to care for patients and constantly-changing guidelines about when exposed and ill frontline workers could return to work."

The internet and media were full of pictures and accounts from frontline workers pleading for people to stay home, as the hospitals were so full they were having to wear garbage bags and other household products makeshifted into PPE to care for the surplus of patients. I myself was reusing a single-use N95 (I still am) as we were told as long as it was not "visibly soiled" it was to be recycled—a stark contrast from decades of education and practice preceding.

Hospitals across the state worked endlessly to find ways to expand while government leaders worked with the Army Corps of Engineers to build field hospitals, such as the one at the Javits Center.

A good snapshot of what occurred in New York is that of Northwell Health, a local regional health care chain with 17 acute-care hospitals. Under normal circumstances, the system ran on 4,000 beds, not including specialized inpatient beds (maternity, psychiatry, etc.). In less than two weeks, the system added 1,500 more beds by utilizing space not typical for general inpatient admission. As the area reached its early April peak of the outbreak, the hospital system had about 5,500 inpatients, of which 3,425 had COVID-19.

Because of such efforts, despite the daily cries for more beds and portrayals of disparity, New York state never ran out of hospital beds.

While some hospitals in the area had to divert care to other local hospitals, initiatives to expand capacity by utilizing existing space and the plummeting demand for non-COVID medical care allowed the state to avoid running out of beds. Not to mention, some of the early estimates regarding hospitalization proved incorrect.

The initial projections calculating the need for hospital beds were based on factors that varied and on assumptions that didn't hold true. Early data from the U.S. Centers for Disease Control and Prevention suggested that for every person who died of COVID-19, more than 11 would be hospitalized, but that changed over time. Initially what was occurring was doctors were admitting more people into the hospital with suspected COVID out of an abundance of caution, rather than ensuring they met admission criteria. As time went on, they got better at admitting only very sick people who needed more aggressive care.

THE VENTILATOR SCRAMBLE

By April 2020, with hospital beds nearly full of patients, breathing machines (ventilators)—along with personal protective equipment (PPE) and tests—were becoming short in supply.

The people who were showing up in the emergency departments with severe symptoms had low blood oxygen levels, what would come to be known as a hallmark of severe COVID-19. Basic protocol historically was that when patients had low blood oxygenation levels, oxygen should be administered. Patients were rapidly placed on oxygen, with many not improving with only face masks and nasal cannulas; physicians therefore placed them on mechanical ventilators to force oxygen into their lungs. The apparent need for mechanical ventilation was occurring much more frequently than with other respiratory illnesses, alarming health care professionals across the world. Also, unlike in normal circumstances, patients with COVID were on ventilators for two to three weeks rather than the average five to seven days, further lessening the supply of available ventilators.

At the beginning of the outbreak, New York's health system had approximately 6,000 ventilators. Back in 2005, the city's health department surveyed the majority of public and private hospitals to gauge potential equipment needs if they were to face a pandemic. The survey found New York's hospitals had roughly 2,700 ventilators back then, significantly less than what would be needed in the event of a severe outbreak. While the city purchased a few thousand additional ventilators in 2006 and 2007, following the release of the pandemic plan, after 2009 the effort to create a large ventilator stockpile dwindled. Cuomo also turned down an opportunity to purchase 16,000 ventilators for the state in 2016; instead he directed the allocated funds toward wind and green energy rebates, as described in an opinion piece by Ross Marchand in early April 2020.

The potential supply-chain issue surfaced again in 2018, when the public hospital system participated in a pandemic exercise with Johns Hopkins University on the one hundredth anniversary of the 1918 flu. The authors published recommendations for New York to improve their response in the event of an outbreak, including restocking depleted supplies.

They knew there would be an equipment shortage in the event of a crunch, so the partisan blame game that emerged was a mere deflection of decades of neglect.

Combining the infection and hospitalization estimates from the earlier projections with the high incidence of hospitalized patients requiring mechanical ventilation, health officials finally started sounding the alarm.

Governor Cuomo told people during a press conference in March that the state needed "at least 30,000 of the breathing machines to care for the influx of coronavirus patients that is expected to hit New York in two weeks."

In response, hospitals again had to put their engineering hats on to find ways to retrofit other equipment to function as ventilators. Additionally, the federal government dispatched ventilators from the stockpile to help with the shortage.

Rather than acknowledging the efforts being made and admitting to decades of inattention, Cuomo chose to politicize the situation by saying the federal government had sent an insufficient number of ventilators and that President Trump should "pick the 26,000 people who are going to die" because they lack ventilators.

But New York never ran out of ventilators and although the exact number has not been published, it can be surmised that if the peak hospitalizations consisted of 18,000 people by mid-spring and during that time the upper end of hospitalized patients requiring ventilation was 33 percent, this would indicate a maximum of 5,940 ventilators were being used at one given time. So, Cuomo saying 26,000 people were going to die because the federal government didn't send enough was grossly incorrect.

Rather than rejoicing in the ability to outfit existing materials to save lives, the partisan blame game of COVID-19 continued to evolve.

Supporters of the Democrats sought to place blame on the Trump administration for not providing more, despite the "more" not ultimately being necessary. Supporters of the Republicans placed blame on the Obama administration for not restoring adequate ventilators in the stockpile and on Democratic leadership in New York State for the lack of funding created by Medicaid expansion.

While the country was fretting about lacking equipment most had never heard of before, physicians and researchers began working to improve their treatment protocols for COVID-19 to further lessen the need for ventilators and to improve the high mortality rate.

Reuters interviewed 30 doctors and medical professionals who treated COVID-19 patients in countries across the world, including the United States, China, Italy, Germany, and Spain. Nearly all noted that there were risks from using mechanical ventilators, from either placing patients on them too early or too frequently, or from doctors not familiar with ventilator-use utilizing them in overwhelmed hospitals.

We might usefully contrast the obsessive concern for randomly controlled research trials required for determining travel bans, mask wearing, and medications with the utter indifference to the question of whether mechanical ventilation had even been proven to be an effective treatment for SARS-CoV-2.

As Norman Doidge, MD, aptly pointed out in *Tablet* magazine, "All the commentators who railed that HCQ [hydroxychloroquine] was 'unproven' because there had been no randomized control trials (RCTs) didn't mention that standard ventilation treatment for COVID-19, which had become treatment-as-usual overnight for severe cases, had no RCTs supporting it either."

In fact, a May 11 *Wall Street Journal* article explained that early aggressive ventilator use led to "worse outcomes," which is why early ventilation became less prevalent as the pandemic went on. But again, no one knew. Nothing nefarious or inept occurred early on. Physicians were scrambling to save lives and followed protocols for other respiratory ailments that required ventilation.

So, it turned out that the dire ventilation shortage was overestimated, but the political warfare introduced the illusion of gross ineptitude of the federal and local governments, and even medical professionals' inability to treat the illness.

Americans were afraid.

President Trump, Governor Cuomo, and everyone around them were blamed for the supposed deficiency of ventilators.

In New York, however, the state by that point had so many ventilators they began donating them to other states.

Yet, while the ventilator needs may have been overestimated initially, New York City area hospitals were squeezed to utilize every square inch to make room for patients that spring.

THE VULNERABLE AMONG US

Early in the pandemic, New York found itself the epicenter of a virus outbreak that threatened to overwhelm hospitals. Removing medically stable patients from hospitals to nursing homes was an initial strategy meant to help hospitals handle the increased number of incoming patients.

However, it was apparent early on that elderly patients and those with underlying comorbidities were being reported across the globe to have a drastically higher fatality rate than younger populations. Countless families and individuals all over the world have since learned in excruciatingly painful detail just how much the elderly and those with existing comorbidities (with obesity being crucial in this context) are vulnerable to SARS-CoV-2.

We should have known. As early as January 2020, it was being reported in Chinese media that "Almost half of the 17 people killed by the Wuhan coronavirus so far were aged 80 or over and most of them had pre-existing health problems, according to China's health authorities."

In an effort to free up hospital beds, several states including New York, New Jersey, and California initiated an order for medically stable COVID-19 patients to go into nursing homes. On March 25, Governor Cuomo's administration formally issued "Advisory: Hospital Discharges and Admissions to Nursing Homes."

The order, in which "NH" refers to "nursing home," stipulated that *"No resident shall be denied re-admission or admission to the NH solely based on a confirmed or suspected diagnosis of COVID-19. Nursing homes are prohibited from requiring a medically stable hospitalized resident to be tested for COVID-19 prior to admission or readmission."* It should also be noted that two days prior to this announcement, on March 23, Governor Cuomo had issued an executive order establishing that

> **all physicians, physician assistants, specialist assistants, nurse practitioners, licensed registered professional nurses and licensed practical nurses shall be immune from civil liability for any injury or death alleged to have been sustained directly as a result of an act or omission by such medical professional in the course of providing medical services in support of the State's response to the COVID-19 outbreak, unless it is established that such injury or death was caused by the gross negligence of such medical professional.**

The joint effect of these directives was that COVID-19 patients going from the hospital to nursing homes were not to be discriminated against, regardless of whether they were still contagious or not. The second part of the order was that the facility, caregivers, and medical personnel alike would have no culpability if any negative consequences of these government-directed actions occurred.

Based on a report from the New York State Department of Health, following the order, "between March 25 and May 8, approximately 6,326 COVID-positive patients were admitted to nursing homes," KHN reported.

While many enjoyed the daily televised updates from Governor Cuomo, likening them to suppertime chats with their Italian grandfathers, what was unfolding in the nursing homes and other long-term care facilities was tragic and deserved less grandstanding.

By early November 2020, the virus infected more than 581,000 people at some 23,000 long-term facilities across the nation.

As 2020 came to an end, the death toll discrepancy between states was readily apparent with respect to nursing homes. In 17 states, at least half of COVID-19 deaths occurred in long-term care patients. Overall from available data, the average fatality rate at long-term care facilities was approximately 16 percent, notably higher than the 2 percent case fatality rate occurring nationwide. The noticeably higher rates prompted inquiries into the sites and mandated edicts, pushing the response measures to undergo review.

For example, Massachusetts, a state that did not follow New York's lead in the nursing home mandate, set aside facilities to care for COVID-19 patients. The New England state even emptied one site of other residents and reopened seven closed facilities to treat positive patients.

While the two states had vastly different responses to their actions, their outcomes surprised many.

Interestingly, in Massachusetts, by late fall 2020, an overwhelming 64 percent of all deaths had been related to nursing homes, with the entire state having only a 6 percent fatality rate. Florida too, also a state without the nursing home order, with an overall fatality rate nearly one-third of New York's, had 40 percent of their deaths being nursing home–related.

Conversely, as *The New York Times* reported in late October 2020, New York's nursing home deaths accounted for the smaller fraction of 20 percent of all New York COVID-19 deaths, one of the lowest percentages across the country. If you were to go off of the data alone, one would imagine New York demonstrated the greatest ability of protecting its most vulnerable during the worst crisis in a century.

If only the story ended there.

You see, New York, unlike other states, decided not to count deaths of nursing home residents that occurred in the hospital.

When this discrepancy in reporting was discovered, Cuomo responded to such claims by saying that "if you died in a nursing home, it's called a nursing home death. If you die in a hospital, it's called a hospital death. It doesn't say where you were before." Also, every time he was questioned about his state's nursing home death toll, he framed the inquiries as being politically motivated, while grandstanding that "his" rates were lower than those of the surrounding states, including Massachusetts. This, despite the fact that they report nursing home deaths differently.

The problem with such a mentality is that it decreases the amount of deaths reported as a result of infections occurring in the nursing home. An administrator at one of New York's nursing homes commented in an interview with the Associated Press that the true number compared to the official state count of just four deaths in its 146-bed facility was "far worse." While only four deaths may have occurred at the home, 21 of their residents had actually died from COVID-19, the majority having been transported to hospitals before they succumbed.

A couple of months after the nursing home mandate was announced, the governor rescinded the order, saying hospitals could no longer discharge patients to the long-term care facilities until they test negative for the virus.

The official nursing home death count at the end of 2020 stood at 7,602 New Yorkers. This number still only includes residents who died inside the nursing home and not those who died after being transferred to hospitals, likely thousands more.

The governor continued to deflect blame onto the federal government. Governor Cuomo insisted that he was following guidance from the Centers for Disease Control and Prevention when issuing the nursing home orders.

The devil is in the details on this one and while some people may accept that reasoning, according to the CDC guidance issued in mid-March there were two factors to consider when decisions were being made about whether to discharge a patient with COVID-19 to a long-term care facility or not: if the patient was medically stable, and whether the facility was capable of implementing the recommended infection-control procedures.

In response to the growing condemnation of the state's action, the New York health department released an analysis reporting that asymptomatic nursing home staffers played a larger role in viral transmission among nursing homes than the over 6,000 recovering COVID-19 patients who were transferred there from the hospitals. Public health experts ridiculed the account for flawed methodology that ignored key questions, including the state's timing of cases and mortality, rather than focusing on contact tracing of patients, staff, and family members.

Ultimately, from a scientific viewpoint, there is an important reason to report how many deaths occurred due to facility-acquired infections. Such information is vital to modeling future preparedness and response protocols for the exposed long-term care facilities.

By September of 2020, the Justice Department was embarking upon an investigation into the nursing home deaths. Despite multiple federal attempts to collect data from New York hospitals and nursing homes, the New York governor evaded responsibility and undermined transparency, knowing that the true number would make "his" nursing home fatality rates much higher. Yet in late November 2020 the governor was awarded an International Emmy for his "masterful" daily televised briefings, despite many of the details he provided during the briefings having proven false. As 2021 began, the cries for transparency and accountability for Governor Cuomo's nursing home decisions were getting louder, suggesting justice for the victims' families might come.

Regrettably, political posturing has caused sidestepping in the quest for truth, and whether we will ever get an accurate death count related to nursing home residents remains unknown. The lack of transparency and potential for negligence have made a tragic situation even more shattering.

If we were to rewind back to before these deaths occurred, one of the most memorable images from the early pandemic is that of the U.S. Navy hospital ship, the USNS *Comfort*, as it sailed into New York Harbor past the Statue of Liberty on the cloudy day of March 30, 2020, to provide 1,000 additional hospital beds and 12 operating rooms.

The arrival of the ship marked one of the few moments for which no one assigned blame. It was a beacon of hope sent to save a suffering populace at the insistence of the governor as the state's hospital capacity was maximized and long-term care facility residents were falling.

Yet, three weeks later, the ship sailed out, having barely been used.

An August 28, 2020, op-ed in *The Wall Street Journal* blasted the Cuomo administration: "Mr. Cuomo continued to send recovering Covid patients back to nursing homes even when there were plenty of surge beds—both in a U.S. Navy hospital ship, and the Javits Center hospital that the Trump Administration built. A Brooklyn nursing home on April 9 asked the state to transfer vulnerable patients to these field hospitals. Mr. Cuomo said no."

Despite New York having multiple makeshift locations to house patients, they largely went unused.

Because of strict visitation restrictions, many elderly residents who had been exposed to the virus suffered alone, uncomforted, with no family members allowed by their side.

We may not have known much about this sickness by the time the virus entered our borders, but we knew the elderly were extremely vulnerable.

The information was there. The resources were there. While some of the initial mishaps can be attributed to evolving evidence regarding the virus, it was clear older populations were the most susceptible to this illness, yet they were not protected the way they should have been.

HISTORY REPEATS ITSELF

Back in 1918, as influenza was raging, the city of Philadelphia notoriously refused to cancel a parade that was scheduled for September 28. The parade was supposed to rally public support for the U.S. efforts in the Great War, and, more specifically, to sell war bonds. This single event led to the largest clustered outbreak in the locale during the pandemic.

Over a century later, on March 3, 2020, New York's Lieutenant Governor Kathy Hochul and Health Commissioner Dr. Howard Zucker joined the New York State American Academy of Pediatrics and over 100 anti-vaping advocates inside the State Capitol to rally support for a ban on vaping products—an honorable cause, but one that should have been canceled as the alarm bells were going off about the evolving epidemic.

The New York Times reported, "Publicly . . . as late as March 9, the Health Department was not recommending the closure of events, like the city's half marathon, according to an email shared with The Times." In an email from Dr. Katz, president and CEO of NYC Health + Hospitals, to Mayor de Blasio on March 10, which was obtained by the *Times*, Katz worried that such shutdowns would cause residents to overestimate the severity of the virus. "Canceling large gatherings gives people the wrong impression of this illness," he wrote. "Many of the events are being canceled anyway, and fewer people are going out. However, it is very different when the government starts telling people to do this." He made a case that fear of the virus was more dangerous than the virus itself.

Philadelphia's director of public health during the 1918 epidemic, Wilmer Krusen, might have been worried about the growing epidemic, given that the flu had already ravaged the Great Lakes region and Boston. But, as John Barry remarks in the book that so impressed President George W. Bush, "Krusen saw [the] reports and heard from those who wanted to cancel the parade, all right, but he didn't seem to be listening." He put a few restrictions in place, and the parade happened as scheduled, with predictable consequences. Two days after the parade, Krusen issued a dismal statement: "The epidemic is now present in the civilian population."

If, back in the summer of 2005, the story of the 1918 pandemic moved an American president to take dramatic action, so too should the still unfolding story of the SARS-CoV-2 pandemic. That the current pandemic happened during a presidential election cycle makes the faulty overlap between science and politics all the more urgent—because, rhetoric notwithstanding, neither political party has a monopoly on science.

CHAPTER 13

PUSHING BACK THE REGULATORY RED TAPE

We had no idea where the virus was spreading in the country.

The lack of the ability to widely test for SARS-CoV-2 left policy-makers, health care workers, and every American facing an invisible enemy. The rapid uptick of patients coming to the emergency departments with flu-like and respiratory symptoms with a negative flu test signaled COVID-19 was here. However, without accessible testing we were left navigating blindly.

The lack of testing was just one thing hampered by the pointless mass of red tape with which we've bound medical professionals.

TESTING

Indisputably, there was no early, aggressive SARS-CoV-2 testing. The pandemic response plans created for such occurrences all assumed diagnostic capability would be available. Had this been another influenza pandemic, it would have been. It seemed the country would have been better equipped to handle a flu pandemic, but this wasn't influenza.

Some of the challenges probably couldn't have been avoided. The Food and Drug Administration had a long-standing practice of preventing academic and other private labs from running their own laboratory-developed tests, and as the novel coronavirus had never been seen before, no test kits were pre-approved for use. The delay can be traced to the administrative state and its attendant regulations requiring such outside labs to undergo intense federal review before utilizing new methods. It is less clear whether either political party or official is to blame in this respect, or that negligence or sinister intent was involved. Perhaps we will lessen those regulations moving forward, but there will always be a price to pay for cutting safety corners; there is a fine line between maintaining quality and reducing oversight.

We also didn't know if we could trust Chinese tests. An administration official noted to me that they had seen preliminary testing data from the Chinese, but it was all speculative. They knew the infection and death rates in China were likely higher than those being reported. Either the test being used in China was flawed, giving false negatives, or they were hiding or possibly lying about the case counts. Thus, the U.S. rejected the test from China under the belief it could not be used with confidence.

But then the first mistake happened. On February 5, 2020, the Centers for Disease Control and Prevention, the nation's preeminent agency for managing public health, hastily released its own SARS-CoV-2 testing kits. Given the timing of their release, the tests met—or seemed at first to meet—an urgent need.

The FDA's regulations compounded this mistake, however.

The Food and Drug Administration restrictions meant that for the first critical weeks, no one outside of the federal government was allowed to independently develop and distribute tests.

This meant the CDC was the sole source for the test kits.

"We're in good hands," a public health official at the CDC involved in the process reassured colleagues by email, according to *The Washington Post.*

Three weeks after the tests were sent out, this confidence proved to be incorrect. Verification tests by public and private laboratories found that they were defective, and their results untrustworthy.

Other tests were available internationally, and various laboratories in the U.S. had also developed prototypes. Yet the FDA refused to alter their approval processes to hasten their review and distribution. A pathologist from the University of Washington said, off the record, that when they urgently submitted a testing application to the FDA in January, immediately following the release of the virus's gene sequence, they were told to fill out a 32-page form. Despite the grueling administrative bloat this brought on the research team, it was done. Unfortunately, it was ultimately rejected because, while the application was done precisely, the files were sent electronically rather than burned onto an archaic CD ROM.

Rejected.

Imagine something so ridiculous being the hindrance for our nation's ability to test at the onset of the pandemic. Unfortunately, the rapidity of government programs accelerating treatments, vaccines, and other technologies didn't occur until later.

In an article in the *MIT Technology Review*, Neel V. Patel noted, "The CDC's kits are based on PCR testing, which makes millions or billions of copies of a DNA sample so that clinicians can easily identify and study it." Patel then asked the necessary question: "So how exactly does the CDC, of all places, goof up something so tried and true?" He rightly pointed out that "PCR is a very sensitive test. You need extremely clean reagents, and the smallest contaminants can ruin it completely (as happened in this instance)." In this case, he noted, the fact that "many of the kits were soon found to have faulty negative controls (what shows up when coronavirus is absent), caused by contaminated reagents . . . was probably a side effect of a rushed job to put the kits together."

The question remains as to why we were so focused on a high-quality PCR test in the first place rather than a less expensive, less sensitive lateral assay rapid test that could have been more widely distributed with fewer supply-chain disturbances. What we needed early on was a screening test to capture more at their highest infectivity rather than a higher-quality (and more expensive), precise diagnostic test. We got neither. This was a major blunder of the pandemic response. Had we been able to efficiently and accurately identify positive cases, subsequent missteps may have been avoided.

Unbelievably, it took three weeks after the failed CDC tests were released before the FDA relented, allowing tests to be used from other sources. On February 29, 2020, the FDA issued a press release confirming that other laboratories would be allowed to develop and distribute test kits for the virus.

Three weeks is an eternity in pandemic time. By the time tests began to be more widely available, the proverbial barn door was wide open and the livestock was romping across the land.

Once the regulations had been changed, the Seattle Flu Study began testing specimens using their own PCR testing for SARS-CoV-2. Unlike the PCR tests from the CDC, these tests worked and began identifying positive cases immediately.

As the country slowly began catching up with testing, our supply chain's reliance on China, India, and various other countries became obvious as reagents and other necessary items were slow to trickle in. Testing capacity was ramping up, but the supply chain shortage stripped our ability to adequately do it.

The failure of widespread testing availability in February and early March ultimately led to the harsh lockdowns, because we did not have situational awareness of the transmission of the virus within the United States.

The inability to test broadly paralyzed the U.S. response at the only point at which the crisis could have realistically been nipped in the bud. Instead of an intense and targeted testing and contact tracing operation, we effectively attempted an unprecedented quarantine of the entire (healthy) population. The costs have been very high.

But who is ultimately to blame for the lack of testing? It is true that the country was prepared for a flu pandemic because it had learned lessons from prior events. However, the U.S. was inexperienced dealing with coronavirus outbreaks, as other countries had been previously. This was a crisis caused by a novel virus for which there was no preexisting test and U.S. officials had reason to believe the tests being utilized elsewhere were substandard. That said, there were plenty of unforced errors caused by having a bloated and inefficient bureaucracy handling the rollout of testing. Inarguably, a substandard test is better than no test, and perhaps that is the lesson to be learned here. Even more, the regulatory red tape restricted development and our testing abilities, leading to a rapid rise in infected people requiring hospitalization. We were desperate for reinforcements, and the emergency requirement was about to expose how pointless and counterproductive so many of our medical regulations are.

TEARING DOWN BARRIERS

Cases continued to rapidly expand throughout the tristate area. Public health officials and hospital administrators were watching the news from Italy showing footage of overwhelmed hospitals and exhausted staff trying desperately to cope. Like in China, Italian frontline workers were falling ill, many dying. The dread of potential consequences burdened the State of New York as it began to prepare.

Perhaps the fears were useful. When push came to shove, and public health experts and policymakers saw there would be terrible penalties for failing to act, a few barriers to commonsense flexibility in the provision of medical care suddenly came down. Just like that, qualified, licensed medical professionals were allowed to treat critically ill patients—even if those sick patients happened to be across state lines. Within record time, hurdles to state licensing and telemedicine restrictions were eliminated. Doctors were allowed to consult with patients over virtual platforms, instead of requiring them to haul themselves in to crowded waiting rooms. These were sensible changes, yet they had been held up in legislative purgatory for years.

The rules that prevented doctors and nurses from treating patients with flexibility in the pre–SARS-CoV-2 era are only a small part of the vast catalogue of regulatory red tape with which medical professionals are bound.

Comprising thousands of pages of legalese, these rules govern almost every detail of interactions between medical practitioners and patients. Digging into the way medical care is delivered, the resemblance to the worst characteristics of centrally controlled economies stands out. That isn't coincidental.

Health care for the most part is externally controlled, although markets are still allowed more scope in the U.S. than in most other places. The reason being, the vast majority of health services is paid for by somebody other than the person who receives it.

And the more expensive medical care gets, the more control is exerted by the people paying for it.

Of course, to control it, they have to know exactly what everyone is doing.

This is why you probably see your doctor typing away on a laptop instead of talking to you.

Payers, government and private alike, want a record of precisely what occurs, so that they can regulate it. Therefore, control over what doctors, nurses, and other medical professionals do requires rules. Lots and lots of rules.

The result—which no one likes—is that doctors who have a good idea of how to help patients often cannot simply do so.

Unfortunately, the hefty regulation means in many circumstances, things that might seem to be appropriate are simply not allowed. And it can be very hard to change the rules. However, a small silver lining of the pandemic has been that hundreds of rules and regulations that were deemed essential in the pre–SARS-CoV-2 era were suddenly swept away. All it took was having a really good reason to do something that made a lot of sense to begin with, but which somehow never got done.

CROSSING STATE LINES

On Friday, April 3, 2020, I received an email and text message simultaneously that on any other day, I would have disregarded as spam and immediately deleted. However, this one caught my eye as it was in ALL CAPS, declaring "ATTENTION all healthcare workers: New York City is seeking licensed healthcare workers to support healthcare facilities in need." It seemed, all physicians who held a license in New York received this alert as a cry for help to fill the void as workers were falling ill caring for infected patients.

Would enough medical professionals respond? With case counts rising, the fear was that there might not be enough qualified volunteers available locally. Responding to the pleas of public health officials and hospital administrators, Governor Andrew Cuomo publicized a national appeal for trained medical professionals to supplement the stretched staff of overloaded hospitals. In an extraordinary outpouring of generosity, tens of thousands of nurses, doctors, EMTs, and other frontline workers from across America responded, offering to travel to New York and help.

No one seemed to seriously pause to think that experienced nurses and doctors who were licensed by states other than New York could not just walk in and help treat patients in New York.

Out the window went the long-protected prerogative of state governments to restrict permission to practice across state lines without undergoing the specific state's licensure process and of course, paying hefty fees. Some states while in pre-COVID had made plans for a potential public health emergency by passing legislation to consider special rules for emergencies under the Uniform Emergency

Volunteer Health Practitioner Act (UEVHPA), allowing the state to recognize out-of-state licenses. But New York state was not one of them. For some reason, New York seemed to be the outlier when we examined many of the details regarding response and preparedness. As the state was low on medical professionals to care for ailing patients, it took emergency declarations to allow physicians and other frontline responders from outside the state to assist.

The urgency of the needs that arose in New York City was a reality check.

In the space of days, detailed rules allowing out-of-state practitioners to legally operate were carefully hammered out by state licensing boards in cooperation with professional organizations to condense down a handful of critical checks to provide needed reinforcements for the struggling staff in New York hospitals.

Over the next few months, public health officials in all 50 states and the District of Columbia went through the same mental calculations and reached similar conclusions, greatly reducing the barriers to practicing medicine. In addition, states appealed to medical and nursing students who had recently graduated but had not yet passed licensing exams, and to retired workers with expired licenses. It was all hands on deck.

My friend and colleague Paul Lynch, an anesthesiologist from Arizona whom I had met while training at the Mayo Clinic, answered the plea. He had spent years of his education in New York City during his residency so he felt compelled to return the favor to the people. He left his wife and children at home as he flew to New York to stay in a small hotel and work endless shifts helping to manage the overflowing ICUs. He chronicled his journey in a series of YouTube videos, including when he himself became ill. While the COVID tests came back negative, he was quarantined in his hotel room with high fevers and all the symptoms of COVID-19, a disease he referred to as "the disease of isolation."

He knew the risk was high coming to the hot zone and with his faith in God and dedication to the medical community within him, he pushed on. After nearly a month of being in New York City, personally intubating numerous patients needing to be placed on a ventilator, he returned safely home to his family and medical practice, where he continued to educate his community on the dangers of COVID-19. It had been decades since his training in New York, so while he was qualified to help during the crisis, had the red tape not been cut to allow him to provide care across state lines, he would never have been able to come.

TELEHEALTH

By this time, people were being told to stay home to lessen the spread. The overriding message was that the only reason to leave your house was for essentials or emergencies. Meanwhile, hospitals and doctors around the country were scrambling to protect their patients. With the constant barrage of information telling people that the elderly and those with chronic medical conditions were most at risk of dying of COVID, the double-edged sword is that this population also tends to require more frequent medical care for various other reasons.

The new problem people were being faced with was, how were these people going to keep access to their doctors while staying safe from COVID-19?

Providing medical care via remote platforms—typically called telehealth—seemed like a no-brainer, even before the pandemic.

Imagine that you live in a rural area where specialists are few and far between. You need to see a specialist and the nearest one is three hours away by car. You can easily have all your test results and imaging delivered electronically, so it is the consultation that historically required an in-person exchange. This can be, of course, exhausting and expensive, particularly for patients who are ill.

Limited rollouts of medical care via telehealth platforms had already happened, but on a very tiny scale, for only a handful of people. To offer telehealth services, providers and insurers faced a bewildering thicket of federal and state regulations on privacy and state licensure, combined with restrictions on reimbursement from both public and private insurers.

Technology had already provided the tools to make this happen, sitting on the shelf, ready to go. It was idly waiting for policymakers to allow its use. The machinery to facilitate remote access to care was waiting to be deployed. The pandemic acted as the catalyst to create the expansion that advocates for telehealth had long fought for.

I myself, because of a chronic autoimmune disease, had already put in for a remote workstation a year before the pandemic struck. As expected, I was told that although approved for such a station, it would likely not be delivered for 12 to 18 months. At the time the urgency was not there to work and connect with patients remotely; however, because of occasional symptom flare-ups and treatment side effects, the option to work from home every now and then was preferable. As SARS-CoV-2 became increasingly present in our community, knowing that I was taking a medication designed to suppress my immune response, my insistence on the workstation intensified. Accepting that the country was in a crisis, I knew the equipment was not a priority at that moment, nor should it have been. Therefore, as I made plans to head into the hospital, when I asked to wear an N95 mask into work, my request was denied as the insistence of universal mask-wearing in hospitals hadn't materialized yet.

Initially the concern was that mask-wearing in nonprocedural settings would incite panic and waste resources, especially if a medical-grade N95 was being worn. As I was scrambling to find ways to care for my patients while also protecting myself, administrative barriers remained. After I forfeited a week of already-limited vacation time, the policy was changed and universal mask wearing was not only allowed but required. Soon to follow was the delivery of the home workstation. I was armed with the equipment needed to continue vital care for my patients while also protecting myself from the virus that we knew little about during the early days of crisis. A robust telehealth system was created and quality, necessary care was delivered. But again, it took a pandemic to push forth actions that should have been done months (probably years) earlier.

In a modest success story of the pandemic, the regulatory and reimbursement walls that had long prevented telehealth from growing beyond a small niche were knocked down in record time.

On March 13, 2020, President Trump issued an emergency declaration in response to the pandemic allowing Medicare to issue waivers to existing rules. Centers for Medicare Services (CMS) wasted no time in using that authority, issuing emergency changes to the rules to expand access by Medicare beneficiaries to care via telehealth. Suddenly, patients could receive medical care remotely, in any location, including in the comfort and safety of their home. The scope of Medicare services that could be provided was also expanded. It was a clear success story for the handling of the virus, as the elderly population most vulnerable to COVID was handed an important lifeline.

Private insurers and state Medicaid authorities followed Medicare's lead and expanded remote access as well.

On balance, it has worked.

So, this achievement has the potential to be the kind of progress made during the pandemic that we might hope for: a boost to the efficiency of medical care and a big help to rural populations and the medically vulnerable. The question that remains is, what happens when the emergency declarations go away?

My hopes are high, but there are some disquieting signs. A report of the Taskforce on Telehealth Policy Findings and Recommendations was released on September 15, 2020. Its recommendations to continue the efforts, while acknowledging successes of telehealth, were weaker than advocates hoped for.

Given the inertia that tends to exist in the state public health authorities where many of the key regulations reside, there is going to be a strong temptation to go back to the status quo once the pandemic is behind us.

On the other hand, telehealth has powerful advocates that it didn't have before. Those advocates are now the patients—patients who are able to access vastly expanded options for qualified doctors, specialists, and therapists, outside of the little room in the office building that has been the only option until now. Somehow, I think those people will make their voices heard.

In fact, it was the will of the people that helped turn the state of calamity in the Northeast around. They only needed to be told how. This is the only way we'll cut through the red tape of regulations and get government working for the people again.

CHAPTER 14

FORK IN THE ROAD

Winners and Losers

Think back on the iconic New York City, the Statue of Liberty, Broadway, Times Square, great food: remember the way it was rather than what it has now become.

For true New Yorkers, a stubborn refusal to leave the city that they love is implicit in their affection for it. They will never leave. But for many now, to think of New York City's Central Park or, indeed, New York City at all, is to think of social breakdown and a perilous threat to one's life and limbs, and the desperation to escape the boarded-up, tattered city.

The damage done to the city by the pandemic has been heavy. It has taken a hefty toll that can be measured empirically in terms of the number of masked people who, in the long, unsettled summer of 2020, stood in socially distanced lines, checking their phones as they waited to rent U-Haul trucks to pack up their things and escape from New York. Reuters reported that in 2020, "A net 70,000 people left the metropolitan region this year, resulting in roughly $34 billion in lost income . . . 3.57 million people left New York City . . . between Jan. 1 and Dec. 7, according to Unacast, which analyzed anonymized cell phone location data. Some 3.5 million people earning lower average incomes moved into the city during that same period." By early September of that year, real estate values in Manhattan and the boroughs were tanking and, correspondingly, people's lives were being disrupted.

Like invasive ivy consuming a landscape, the virus spread throughout the tristate area's congested indoor spaces and over-crowded public transportation systems before making its way across the rest of the country. It did this just as college students headed off for warm-weather spring break destinations and families absconded, attempting to escape the virus in sunny Florida and elsewhere across the country.

We have already seen the extent to which efforts to slow the spread of a virus are complicated by the simple problem that, during a pandemic, people don't want to stay put. Where they go, the virus goes with them from house to house, town to town, and state to state.

Once the virus was well-established within the U.S., differences between state governments came into play. While the federal government has the authority to order a quarantine to prevent the introduction, transmission, and spread of communicable diseases from foreign countries into the United States, the states are responsible for enacting statutes for quarantine within their boundaries.

Immediate measures to limit domestic travel, such as interstate travel restrictions, may have delayed widespread transmission. Yet domestic travel restrictions, like international ones, are equally controversial, with economic implications and may be unlikely to reduce the impact that the pandemic has on any one community over the long term.

The issue requires balancing two opposite effects of uncertain scale: on the one hand, the benefits in terms of slowing COVID-19 contagion to allow the hospital system to accommodate and save lives; on the other hand, the potential for harm to the economy and to people's long-term health and livelihoods.

The way COVID-19 has become politicized—with partisan divides on a broad variety of issues, including mask-wearing, stay-at-home orders, and whether the pandemic itself is a myth—has meant some governments have made decisions that fly in the face of empiricism rather than logical rationalism.

Although the United States leads the world in many facets, when it came to responding to the pandemic, we are proving mediocre at best. We certainly know a lot more about how to handle this disease than we did to begin with. And after all, learning from experience is what propels a nation forward. Could we have done better? Of course. The example of Sweden offers an example of how voluntary measures and reasonable restrictions can help avoid some of the social and economic problems associated with harsh lockdowns, though it also doesn't eliminate all problems.

SWEDEN

In stark contrast to the United States, Sweden stood out as a country focused on a contrarian approach, an outcast to surrounding nations and most of the rest of the world by not implementing harsh lockdown orders early in the pandemic. Sweden's seemingly laissez-faire approach to the coronavirus provoked a partisan response, with one side hailing their individualistic method of protecting the greater good of the country while critics grew angrier by the day.

Like anti-Trumpers who refuse to acknowledge any progress from the administration whether it is the economy, low unemployment, or even the rapid advancements of vaccines during a global crisis, lockdown enthusiasts determinedly filter out the favorable aspects of the Swedish response. Contrarily, those opposed to the lockdowns and closures were demanding the United States adopt Sweden's measures.

Most of the changes in Sweden involved voluntary actions by citizens, rather than restrictions imposed by the government. While their testing remained less per capita than most of the rest of the world (which may have falsely lowered infection numbers), those infected were tasked with doing their own contact tracing and quarantines.

Over the course of the spring months, as with the United States, nursing home deaths were overwhelming, but once the elderly were identified as vulnerable and protections were put in place, the deaths slowed.

While the Swedes benefited from less economic fallout than the remaining Eurozone, a measure of their success is that they seemingly avoided the hostile fervor and dread that has overtaken our society. They had cases, they had death, but they didn't have the panic imposed by stay-at-home orders.

So were they right?

Though the early months showed some hope that their method was working with a lower infection rate, by the end of 2020, Sweden was reporting a mortality rate of 57 deaths for every 100,000 residents, according to Johns Hopkins University. This was far higher than the rates of its Nordic counterparts, including Denmark (11) and Norway (5). To compare, the United States at the same time was reporting a mortality rate of 50 deaths for every 100,000 residents.

While the goal was to achieve herd immunity naturally to avoid a second wave in the fall and winter season, the country was nowhere near the threshold as the autumnal equinox approached. As the seasons changed, Sweden began seeing higher levels of infection than the surrounding countries.

After nearly a year of voluntarily managing their crisis and maintaining a smidgeon of normalcy, the second wave of infections began causing rising hospitalizations and deaths. The mounting numbers ultimately led to restrictions including a ban on large gatherings, limits on alcohol sales, and school closures.

There is little comfort and utility in comparing countries in their response and outcomes at this point, as all countries are in a different phase of the pandemic with many variables influencing each measurable data point. But we can look at actions to determine what has worked, what has not, and what we will do the next time a pandemic comes, because we know it will.

To be fair, Sweden cannot be compared to the entire United States in terms of population and cultural diversity, maybe just to South Dakota, which was reporting 107 deaths per 100,000 people at the end of 2020, according to Johns Hopkins data.

So, with similar populations and demographics, how is South Dakota experiencing over twice as many deaths per capita as Sweden when it too was known for not imposing strict measures and mask mandates?

The largest misconception about Sweden, which has been popularized in the United States, is that although the nation may not have instituted strict mandates initially, they didn't have a free-for-all either.

In addition to not requiring face masks, South Dakota welcomed hundreds of thousands of visitors for a massive motorcycle rally over the summer, while also allowing the large state fair to take place. The following weeks and months saw the highest rise in cases, hospitalizations, and deaths per capita across the entire country.

In Sweden, rather than mandates and oppressive closures like elsewhere in the world, recommendations were made to the public to lessen gatherings, work from home, and protect the elderly. While restaurants were not closed, people were dining out less frequently. Schools were also kept in session, while social gatherings and indoor activities decreased. The Associated Press reported:

> This trust given to the population to shoulder personal responsibility in the pandemic puts Sweden at odds with most other countries that used coercive measures such as fines to force compliance.
>
> This is often attributed to a Swedish model of governance, where large public authorities comprised of experts develop and recommend measures that the smaller ministries are ex-

pected to follow. In other words, the people trust the experts and scientists to develop reasonable policies, and the government trusts the people to follow the guidelines.

Generalized mask-wearing was also not adopted. Should it have been? *The Washington Post* pointed out that Sweden is "a country the size of California with only a quarter of that state's population and low levels of transmission," so "most Swedes believe wearing masks makes little sense." Scientifically speaking, it would seem the densely populated areas, such as large cities, utilizing public transit and small indoor spaces may benefit from mask-wearing, but how much science is behind wearing a mask in sparsely populated areas when not in confined quarters? None.

As a contrast, in the United States a person walking alone on a path in the middle of Central Park without a mask on would be subject to verbal criticism and a fine for not covering their nose and mouth. It would seem Sweden was following the science better than we were in some respects, as angry as that may make some people.

But as we see, while Sweden didn't come out as a winner in terms of deaths per capita, they also aren't a loser when one factors in the months of avoiding panic, social unrest, missed childhood education, and severe economic fallout.

When putting into context the Swedish method compared with that of the United States, the Swedes focused on SARS-CoV-2 policy that did not only consider the virus but gave thought to the rest of human life.

Emerging scientific evidence will always have shades of gray, with sequential studies proving and disproving the science of the preceding one.

When we look to New York, a state with some of the strictest measures taken for the longest time during the course of the pandemic, while they could relish the low viral transmission throughout the summer and late 2020, millions have become unemployed, with New York City reporting over a 10 percent unemployment rate. As an estimated half-million people fled the city by the summer, nearly two-thirds of New York restaurants closed permanently by January 2021, and the lights of Broadway remain dark through spring 2021.

Those who could afford to do so went to warmer, less-condensed environments with fewer restrictions. All the while, the poor and newly unemployed were left in a ghost town with little resources and opportunity.

In contrast, sunny Florida reopened the state following summer closures without restrictions or mask mandates. The summer cases in Florida resulting in closures were largely from travelers escaping the Northeast and bringing the virus with them. As the fall and winter months approached, while they saw a rise in cases, their counts did not compare to some of the harder-hit areas of the country. The warm weather continually allowed outdoor activity as many people were distancing and wearing masks of their own volition. Apart from the Orlando area, which is heavily dependent on Disney travel, the state as a whole managed to keep businesses open.

By early March 2021, New York reported 245 deaths per 100,000 while Florida reported 146. It can be argued that New York was hit early, before treatments were available, but both New York and Florida suffered from early infections in the spring. By contrast, California avoided the initial wave, yet strict measures in the later months still resulted in 135 deaths per 100,000.

We now know a lot more about what we should have done to be ready when this pandemic landed on our shores. We lost crucial reaction time because of misinformation. Next time, we can leverage this experience to do things better.

We do not need to reinvent the wheel to ward off pandemics in the future. We need, rather, to heed the lessons of history and experience.

The global pandemic has been an unprecedented shock to the country and to the world.

Placing fault on a single entity for failures to control the novel coronavirus is like blaming someone who has been cemented and dropped in the Hudson River for failing to swim. However, there were key American institutions that had a failure of systemic memory, so the pandemic caught them off guard.

When we compare the United States to other countries, it is essential to look at the timeline. The key differences between the United States and countries such as South Korea, Germany, and New Zealand is that they had high levels of surveillance up and running early on.

People are much better at responding to threats that keep coming at them every day than they are at remaining vigilant against a large, known threat that gets talked about but then fades into the background. Necessity forces us into action.

Even Drs. Fauci and Giroir discussed systemic memory during a Senate hearing in June 2020 as being necessary in order to have a coordinated response and stockpiles for future pandemics and outbreaks. However, unlike most of us, those two should have had systemic memory, as they were both part of the teams involved in the HIV, flu, and Ebola outbreaks.

Early in the pandemic, no one in the United States was especially worried, apart from some who made pleas for caution, and nothing happened. We were complacent. It was a little like the boy who cried wolf, except that the cries were very muted. The wolf, however, was real all along—he just hadn't landed on our doorstep.

Public health authorities in other countries had seen this scenario before. They were ready to act right away, at the point when it actually had the potential to make a difference.

In the United States, SARS-CoV-2 seemed so far away as to be almost off the radar. Remember that even Dr. Fauci saw the risk as minimal in February, while Representative Nancy Pelosi and Mayor Bill de Blasio were sending people out to restaurants and into the streets, encouraging them to visit Chinatown to avoid xenophobia.

The many nations that have done better than the United States at containing the spread and saving lives have done so by two main methods: either by shutting down borders or by implementing tyrannical means to forcibly restrict movement. Interestingly, while the concept of closing borders was immediately disparaged by many within our nation, there seems to be a growing plea within the United States from the same people who also seemingly support more authoritarian policies, a concept that Americans have historically rebuked.

The situation of COVID-19 is complex. Economists and scientists will hardly agree on the best path forward, and what may be justified in one state may not be the best path forward in another as they experience the crisis on different timelines.

While the failures experienced were understandable, they are not excusable.

Action needs to be taken to make sure that the lessons of this pandemic are taken seriously.

Dr. Fauci referred to the pandemic as his "worst nightmare."

This pandemic is a nightmare. However, a color-filled sunrise always follows the darkest of nights. The world's worst pandemic in over a century has a silver lining for Americans: streamlined state and federal bureaucracies, which have given doctors like me greater ability to improve our patients' health and even save their lives.

We may be quick to judge and dismiss those, such as Dr. Fauci, who issue changing recommendations. We may be massively frustrated by elected officials who refuse to bend despite growing pleas for it, as well as credentialed professionals, such as those at the CDC and WHO, who seem not to take into account factors other than the virus. As with every major event in the course of human affairs, people have displayed the usual mix of shortsightedness.

We do not lack for heroes, from the whistleblowers in China to the frontline workers across the globe. We also don't lack for foes, including biased researchers and politicians who impose anti-science measures on the population while not adhering to their own rules.

As for most Americans, perhaps we might reflect upon or, in some cases, admit to ourselves that we wish there were a cleaner line between politics and science. Or wish science was about certainty rather than the disorganized, constantly evolving, continual quest for knowledge.

It would be so helpful in forming our opinions if there were clear sides: one pro-science and one anti-science. There are not. Let's stop projecting fantasies of a battle between ignorant and deluded conservatives on the one hand and righteous, liberal elites on the other.

Legislators and experts alike are tasked to calibrate their responses as the facts on the ground change. The crude partisan narratives suggesting that red states are open collective graves and blue states, by contrast, are humming right along safely is little more than a fiction that is unsupported by reliable data.

Unfortunately, it took far too long for leaders to loosen their grasp and not only entrust people to make decisions for themselves but actually "follow the science."

As we witness shifts in the collective consciousness of our country and chaos, the country is wondering, when will this all end? Everyone is left in a state of panic, asking themselves: what kind of nation have we become and will we be okay?

While the effects of this crisis will be present for years to come, we can confidently know that we are on the path to recovery with the worst far behind us. It is time to take off the politically polarized glasses and rather than looking at the scenario as a Republican or Democrat, or pro-science versus anti-science, see that there is a common path forward for us all, and we are on it together.

AFTERWORD

Writing a book about a crisis while it is still unfolding has certainly had its challenges. Every day some new event adds another question to address or problem to resolve in terms of building up our shared understanding of what to think and how to act as individuals and as members of communities.

The novel coronavirus moves faster than science, largely because scientific progress relies on trial and error while also filtering collective professional judgment and navigating regulatory safeguards. But the process of getting this book—or indeed, any book—to the point that it reaches readers is even slower than science.

By the time that you read these words, much will surely have changed from the time in which they were written. Having said that, there are some things I feel confident will *not* have changed. Most importantly, I want to emphasize that science as such, to the extent that we can generalize about it, does not reflect or respect affiliation with American political parties.

Ultimately, medical science is concerned with nature, not the partisan disputes and factions of the present moment. *There is no "party of science" in this context.* There is certainly no shortage of people choosing their own anti-science narratives, whether to "lock it all down" or "open it all up," to beat up their political opponents or to reinforce social hierarchies. There is, however, a great difference between those who try to absorb scientifically informed knowledge and to act upon it for the sake of preserving their own health and that of others. There will also always be some who believe organized science itself is a conspiracy of sorts and are skeptical of government policies based on it.

Perhaps we would all have more respect for the elite tribes touting recommendations if they were to acknowledge the negative consequences of such actions as well as discuss contrarian beliefs, rather than deflecting blame and censoring them.

An inverse correlation exists between taking science seriously and becoming a sycophant. That is why this book has sought first, to distinguish between science and politics; secondly, to show why we should be wary about mixing them; thirdly, to sift through competing claims and narratives about the novel coronavirus; and lastly, to bring scientifically informed reason, common sense, and, it is to be hoped, some measure of calm to bear upon pandemic-related panic.

Panic can be energizing. Like individual panic attacks, collective panic can release the social equivalent of adrenaline. Panic may give us the need and energy to yell at each other or express our fear and anger in destructive ways. But it leaves us with nothing but wreckage. Once we panic, we seek relief from the distress that it causes, and the relief that we obtain may leave us worse off than we were before it all began.

Panic incites a dependence on the state, a danger that Alexander Hamilton warned about. Do we wish to remain a society capable of establishing good government from internal reflection and choice or are we destined to become dependent on the government's ambitions and force?

In this book, we have laid out information to provide alternatives to panic in the form of facts, knowledge, and the exercise of informed judgment. Certainty is what we want and need. This craving is natural and understandable, but like most cravings, it needs to be controlled. I can't offer certainty, and neither can most of the emerging scientific data on the novel coronavirus.

In the movie *Groundhog Day*, the character played by Bill Murray finds himself in a very strange situation. After the panic of being trapped in a repeating day sets in, he tries over and over to control the situation and to manipulate it for his own benefit. He can't. He ends up becoming miserable, because he doesn't have the inner resources and practical habits that he needs to navigate his strange new reality. Ultimately, he undertakes the hard work of developing new skills, habits, and resources. He adapts and starts working on improving himself in a way that benefits others.

Life, of course, is not a movie, for better or worse. One of the lessons of this pandemic is that some of our most cherished fantasies—including the fantasy that we should all be living in dense urban environments and encouraging global travel under all circumstances—hold dangers as well as possibilities. We have found out the hard way that globalization and urbanization, attractive though they may be for many reasons, hold considerable public health risks.

The damage done by this pandemic has exacted a horrific toll in ruined and lost lives. We have to make something out of it, however, and find new ways to thrive as individuals, members of communities, and citizens. Framing the pandemic in terms of party politics does not improve our chances of thriving.

What does?

We don't need to reinvent the wheel here. As always, taking responsibility for our individual actions, getting informed in such a way that we can promote public health, and listening to people with whom we disagree are more likely to help us achieve our goals than seeking magical cures, trying our darnedest to align our personal political preferences with a mythic notion of "The Science," and demonizing people who hold different views. On an institutional level, our public health agencies and our health care policies more generally need major reform.

While questions still remain as to the origin of the virus, and whether nefarious concealment efforts occurred between the CCP and WHO, the world is at an impasse and must acknowledge that the answers may not reveal themselves for years to come, if ever. What is here now is the real million-dollar question: what has America learned during the course of the pandemic to protect future American lives and the overall health of the country?

Back in the introduction, I noted that the virus is the villain and we should spend less time focusing on fighting with each other rather than fighting the actual virus. That doesn't mean we can't assess the human errors, misjudgments, and acts of negligence—notably, lack of transparency, the dissemination of false information and shoddy data—that have played a role at every stage of this pandemic.

While we can acknowledge the missteps, of course, there has also been tremendous and inspiring heroism in every American that cannot be forgotten.

Fred Rogers—"Mr. Rogers"—famously once remarked, "When I was a boy and I would see scary things in the news, my mother would say to me, 'Look for the helpers. You will always find people who are helping.'" Anyone can criticize or demonize someone else—that is the easy thing to do in times of panic. In the midst of crises, though, we can choose to do the hard but rewarding work of helping others—and ourselves—by working together toward a unified goal, being tolerant of evolving information, and considering those who may not agree with us.

ACKNOWLEDGMENTS

We will all look back on the COVID-19 pandemic and remember the cadre of individuals that became essential to our survival, mentally and physically.

Thank you to Hannah and Eric for making the publishing process appropriately meticulous, transforming words on a page into pages with purpose. Suzanne, for tolerating my flight of ideas and helping put my work into a readable and accurate narrative.

Many thanks to my parents, Becky and Mark, and my siblings, Breanna and Israel, for your love and support despite being 3,000 miles away, without our usual visits.

Thank you to my husband, Paul, and our children, Nicholas, Hudson, and Harrison, for being my constant companions during lockdowns and the year of isolation.

My gratitude to those that made up my small COVID bubble:

- Marty Makary, always a phone call away to decipher data.
- Suzanne, Lauren, Gavin, and Jay, for providing a platform to spread the truth on COVID-19.
- Molly and Kristin, Memorial Sloan Kettering Cancer Center teammates.
- Jennifer and Patrick, indispensable neighbors.
- Nikki and Chet, playdate partners.
- Stacey and Anthony, a constant source of laughter.

INDEX

ABOUT THE AUTHOR

National bestselling author for her first book, *Make America Healthy Again*, Nicole Saphier is a known medical contributor and regular guest anchor for the Fox News Channel. Dr. Saphier is a full-time practicing, board-certified physician at Memorial Sloan Kettering Cancer Center in New York City.